HOARDING DISORDER HELP

15 MINIMALIST STEPS TO HELP YOU DECLUTTER

MILTON HARRISON

© Copyright 2020 - All rights reserved.

It is not legal to reproduce, duplicate, or transmit any part of this document in either electronic means or in printed format. Recording of this publication is strictly prohibited and any storage of this document is not allowed unless with written permission from the publisher except for the use of brief quotations in a book review.

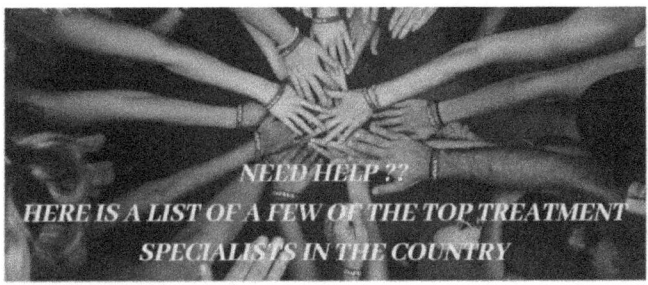

NEED HELP ??
HERE IS A LIST OF A FEW OF THE TOP TREATMENT SPECIALISTS IN THE COUNTRY

THE LIST INCLUDES:

- *Nationally renowned treatment providers*
- *One-click linked portal access*
- *Locations and contact information*
- *Things to remember when seeking or providing help*

It's one thing to need help, and another to know where to go......

To receive your Renowned Treatment List, visit the link:

Renowned Treatment List

CONTENTS

Introduction	7
Step 1: Understanding How Hoarding Disorder Affects You	11
Step 2: Recognizing the Importance of Ongoing Help and Support	26
Step 3: Take Control Through Goal-Setting and Planning	35
Step 4: Design a Schedule and Make Friends With Time	43
Step 5: Create a Sorting System and Prepare Your Resources	48
Step 6: Tackle One Small Area at a Time	53
Step 7: Erase the Maybe - Ask Yourself Questions	59
Step 8: Have a Solid Strategy for When You're Not Sure	66
Step 9: Scale Down Your Collections	75
Step 10: Be Ruthless and Start Again	81
Step 11: Find an Alternative Way to Keep Memories	89
Step 12: Channel Your Need for Control Into Labeling And Organizing	97
Step 13: A Final Clean	104
Step 14: Have a Plan for Staying on Top of the Clutter	112
Step 15: Continue Your Therapy and Use Your Support Network	120
Final Words	129
References	135

INTRODUCTION

"Sometimes letting things go is an act of far greater power than defending or hanging on."

— ECKHART TOLLE

If you are, or if you know, someone who has difficulty parting with literally anything and whose house is so full of clutter that it's nearly impossible to walk through, then it is quite likely the problem is a hoarding disorder. Hoarding disorder is defined as having an ongoing difficulty discarding or parting with possessions because of a perception that it is vital to save them (American Psychiatric Association, n.d.). In fact, just the thought of throwing things away can cause a hoarder significant distress. It's a real disorder that causes emotional pain and social embarrassment.

There are two things, however, to be aware of with this serious condition: First, hoarding disorder is a condition that affects millions of people. Between 2 and 5 percent of US adults suffer from this diagnosis, and up to 5 percent of the global population displays symptoms of hoarding (The Recovery Village, 2020). It's so easy for someone to think they are the only one in the world who feels this way or accumulates so much stuff, but that is far from true. Additionally, this disorder makes sufferers feel as if they are out of control of their environment. They feel helpless in the face of the clutter, and they feel ashamed, which often prevents them from seeking the help they so desperately need. But, the second thing that is important to understand about hoarding is that there is help.

To combat this serious disorder requires a solid plan for helping those affected take back control of their life. It's a process that entails manageable goals and the recognition that relief will not come all at once. It is imperative to take it one step--that is, one manageable goal--at a time. That helps better prepare them emotionally and mentally for the decluttering process. But, if you suffer from this disorder or want to help a loved one who does, where do you start? That's where my professional experience can help.

I received my doctoral degree in psychology from the University of Iowa, and I originally specialized in substance abuse. I became interested in obsessive-compulsive disorder (OCD) after my research showed an overlap between substance abuse and OCD. That led me to become a registered therapist specializing in hoarding disorder and OCD. In fact, as a clinical researcher, I have received funding from the National Institute of Mental Health to conduct research, and from that research, I have published over 150 professional, i.e., peer-reviewed, publications and book chapters on the subjects of substance abuse, OCD, and hoarding disorder. I have also worked as a consultant for hoarding task forces. Additionally, I have given lectures on the overlap between

OCD and substance abuse at universities across the United States. As a result of my professional studies, I have developed a step-by-step guide to help take back control over their lives. This method is highly effective for helping any hoarder declutter their environment.

This book provides you with the tools you'll need to help yourself--or the person affected by hoarding disorder you love--to regain control and understand this challenging condition. The book describes fifteen easy-to-follow, proven steps to take to help hoarders through the declutter process. In fact, here are some of the things you'll discover in the chapters of this book:

- The #1 reason cleaning feels so difficult to do;
- How to construct a plan for decluttering success;
- How it's possible to both keep and get rid of things at the same time;
- Proven tips for managing anxiety;
- The secret to avoiding a relapse,
- How to process those feelings of shame and guilt.

And, there's more. In fact, by using the fifteen steps described in this book, it's possible to clear out as much as 80 percent of the items in the home with very little anxiety. The secrets revealed in this book provide compassionate and effective guidance to help even the most obsessive hoarder get their behaviors in check. Lastly, because everyone is their own worst critic, this book will help anyone who suffers from this condition understand the roots of hoarding and effectively declutter their environment while at the same time learning to treat themselves with compassion and patience.

You, or the loved one you watch suffer with this condition,

no longer have to be ashamed of it. There is help to conquer this disorder once and for all, and you will find it in the pages of this book. The hoarding struggle is an identified disorder by professional psychologists and therapists. And, therapy does work. In fact, as much as 70 percent of patients experience positive results from therapy and are able to get their lives back on track. With the right tools, anyone can overcome this condition. It takes some time, some patience, some compassion, and a good plan. In other words, a clear strategy to take back control and rid yourself from this truly debilitating disorder. Over the course of my professional career, I have seen many success stories. I know it's possible for anyone to benefit from treatment, and I know the guidance I am providing here can help you or your loved one. I have dedicated my life to helping people with hoarding disorder reclaim their lives, and it is my sincere desire to do the same for you. There's no better time than the present to get started on your journey of healing.

STEP 1: UNDERSTANDING HOW HOARDING DISORDER AFFECTS YOU

It's vital to understand the effects of hoarding disorder in order to effectively treat the condition. This overview will help explain hoarding, including the symptoms and effects, which will be helpful for identifying the disorder. The first step to successfully decluttering a home is to recognize the condition and make the decision to seek help. Here are a few of the basics to get a better understanding of hoarding disorder.

Definition of Hoarding Disorder

A hoarding disorder is identified by the acquisition of an excessive number of items which are stored chaotically in a manner that usually results in unmanageable, and often dangerous, amounts of clutter. Additionally, the items are typically of little or no monetary value.

When Does Hoarding Become a Problem?

When the clutter reaches the point where it is interfering with everyday life--for example, the person cannot get to their kitchen--or if the clutter is negatively affecting the individual's quality of life or their family's quality of life, then it has become a significant problem. An example of the latter would be if attempts to clear the clutter create significant distress and affects the familial relationships. If an individual experiences anxiety just at the thought of decluttering a space in their home, then it is interfering with their quality of life. Additionally, if family members attempt to declutter the space, the affected person may become upset, and that can cause problems with their family members. These are signals that this is more than a case of someone being a slob. If there is emotional attachment to the clutter, that indicates a hoarding disorder.

Why is Hoarding So Difficult to Treat?

One of the biggest reasons that hoarding disorder is so difficult to treat is that people often don't even realize they have a problem. They frequently have very little awareness of how their behavior is affecting their life or the lives of their loved ones. Additionally, it's common for hoarders to feel shame, and that can prevent them from seeking help. Because hoarding can result in loneliness and other mental health problems, it's extremely important to encourage them to seek help, because without it, it's quite likely the problem won't resolve itself. And, it can get to the point that it poses a health and safety risk.

What Causes Hoarding Disorder?

Science has yet to fully understand the reasons why someone begins to hoard. It can be associated with other problems. For example, there is evidence that it is associated with obsessive-compulsive disorder (OCD) and obsessive-compulsive personality disorder (OCPD). It may begin with compulsive buying, the compulsive desire to get "freebies," and/or the compulsive search for perfect items. There is also evidence it is associated with severe depression, psychotic disorders such as schizophrenia, and other problems such as attention-deficit/hyperactivity disorder (ADHD). But, it could also be related to something as simple as another illness that prevents the individual from clearing out the clutter they've acquired. If, for example, someone has mobility problems and can't physically remove clutter, then it can accumulate to the point where it becomes overwhelming. Additionally, people with learning disabilities and dementia may not be able to examine the clutter, organize and categorize it, and dispose of those items they no longer need. Their condition may prevent them from being able to do those kinds of mental exercises.

Research (Tolin et al., 2018) also indicates that cognitive impairment is associated with hoarding behaviors. In one study of 83 patients diagnosed with hoarding disorder as compared to 46 healthy control participants, diagnostic interviews and measures of subjective cognitive functioning indicated that the hoarding group demonstrated more impairment than the control group. Furthermore, the degree of cognitive impairment was correlated with the severity of saving and acquiring behaviors. Cognitive impairment was further correlated with the desire to save objects in order to avoid forgetting. These results support current models that indicate decision-making deficits are at the root of hoarding behavior. Cognitive impairment disrupts decision-making skills.

Further research (Grisham & Baldwin, 2015) has sought to understand the neuropsychological underpinnings associated with hoarding disorder. Individuals who suffer from this condition are frequently reported as being easily distracted. This interferes with their ability to manage clutter through organization and by staying on task. This attention deficit was confirmed in research that examined the association of the disorder with attention deficit hyperactivity disorder (ADHD). The results of initial research were confirmed in subsequent studies, which showed more ADHD symptoms in individuals with a hoarding disorder diagnosis as compared to those participants who were healthy and those with anxiety and mood disorders. Still, other research found that those individuals with both OCD and hoarding also had symptoms of ADHD, significantly more so than those OCD patients without hoarding disorder. In those studies using neuropsychological tests to ascertain attention deficits in individuals with hoarding disorder, hoarders were found to have more difficulties than the control group with sustained and spatial attention. Though more research is necessary, there appears to be evidence for deficits in attention among hoarders.

Other research has focused on hoarders' reported desire to keep possessions in order to avoid forgetting them (Grisham & Baldwin, 2015). In fact, concern about memory was shown to be one of the strongest predictors of hoarding behavior in one study. Several studies have found that hoarders have more concern about and poorer confidence in their ability to remember the events and people in their lives. They also tend to overestimate the negative consequences of forgetting. Thus, remembering is a major concern among hoarders. But, does the research bear out their fears? In those studies of laboratory tests of memory, hoarders were, in fact, impaired in their ability to recall and copy organization on a complex figure test as compared to healthy control group participants. Hoarders also were found to have more difficulty with retaining verbal information. These results appear to offer evidence for verbal and visual memory deficits among hoarders. That strongly suggests there may be an association between memory deficits and hoarding.

Still other studies have focused on deficits in executive functioning among hoarders. Executive functioning refers to the ability of an individual to plan and make decisions. Individuals with deficits in executive functioning would have problems discarding and organizing possessions. Impairments in this regard could also be an underlying factor for poor self-regulation that is seen in those individuals with hoarding disorder. That leads to poor self-care and interpersonal deficits. As compared with OCD patients without hoarding, those with hoarding symptoms have been demonstrated to have more difficulty with initiating and completing tasks and problems associated with indecision. It's possible that task-related anxiety is interfering with these results, but hoarding patients do report difficulties in planning and executing complex, strategic motor responses and controlling interference in their efforts. That suggests problems related to self-regulation as expressed by their inability to suppress responses stimulated by a particular environment--for example, a store stimulates the need to acquire and save objects. Problems sustaining motivation for carrying out various tasks, such as discarding unused items, also reflects deficits in self-regulation. One study did find that hoarders experienced impaired decision-making abilities relative to non-hoarders, but that study was not able to be replicated. That may be due to study samples that utilize individuals with both OCD and hoarding as opposed to strictly diagnosed hoarders (Grisham & Baldwin, 2015).

Other research has examined the difficulties that hoarders have with categorization. To efficiently categorize objects, it is necessary to plan, develop grouping strategies, and make decisions related to the placement of objects in a group.

Some research indicates that hoarders have a tendency to create too many, small categories, which ultimately contributes to disorganization and clutter. Hoarding participants in three studies were asked to sort personal and non-personal items into categories. The time to completion for the sorting task, the number of categories created, and the distress experienced by the participant were all measured. When compared with healthy control groups, hoarders created more piles, took longer to sort the items, and reported more distress during the process. All three investigations reported similar findings. Although there were minor discrepancies between the studies, they all support the clinical observations that hoarders have difficulty categorizing items relative to non-hoarding individuals (Grisham & Baldwin, 2015).

It's also possible that hoarding is a condition in and of itself. It is frequently associated with self-neglect. This is reflected in the fact that hoarders are more likely to live alone, be single, have experienced a neglectful or deprived childhood-- i.e., they didn't have very many material things as a child or they had poor relationships with family members-- and/or have a family history of hoarding, which makes them see the clutter as normal. In the latter case, they would never have learned how to declutter; they were never taught how to prioritize and sort items in order to dispose of things they no longer need.

How Do Hoarders Perceive Their Clutter?

Many hoarders have very strong beliefs related to the need for the items they are accumulating. They might believe they will need them someday or that the item is irreplaceable for some reason. They may also associate the possession of an item with happiness or fulfillment. For that reason, any attempt to discard something can generate very strong emotions to the point where the person feels overwhelmed. That prevents them from decluttering--they simply continue to put it off or avoid actually making a decision about what can be discarded. It's also typical that the items in question are of little or no monetary value, something most people would consider rubbish. But, those afflicted with this disorder may claim these items have sentimental value or they're simply beautiful. In fact, many times they will form a strong emotional attachment to the object.

Research has shown that emotional attachments to objects is a key component of hoarding disorder. And, studies have shown that the object attachment experienced by the hoarder represents an attempt to compensate for unmet needs related to social connections. In a sample of 91 undergraduates with hoarding symptoms, object attachment was demonstrated to mediate the relationship between loneliness and hoarding behavior. And, that mediation remained consistent despite adjustments made for age and depression. That suggests that addressing issues of those unmet social connections can help lower object attachment and hoarding symptoms (Yap et al., 2020). This study highlights the importance of therapy in addressing hoarding behavior.

How Does Hoarding Differ from Collecting?

Lots of people collect things, like stamps, coins, or books, and no one thinks of them as hoarders, so what is the difference? The difference really lies in how the items are organized. Most collectors keep their collection well-organized and easily accessible. Hoarders, on the other hand, are very disorganized in their storage of the items they accumulate, and the clutter makes them largely inaccessible. For example, a collector might put newspaper clippings in a scrapbook and catalog them according to subject or time period. In contrast, a hoarder will keep large stacks of newspapers piled up throughout their entire house, which renders any specific item of interest inaccessible. The following descriptions give a better indication of the differences:

- **Collectors**: These individuals have a genuine passion for their subject of their interest. This might be stamps, antiques, model cars, and collectibles. Generally speaking, these individuals form part of a community of people with similar passions and interests. They are not isolated in their interest. They also tend to organize their collections and display them proudly for other people to see.
- **Hoarding**: In contract, because of their inability to organize their clutter, hoarders are not able to display the objects they have collected. Instead, the objects are piled up in their home in such a manner that it is difficult to find anything or even get around. Entryways are either entirely or partially blocked, and navigating from one room to another becomes difficult at best. The objects that hoarders collect also tend to have little monetary value, but despite that fact, hoarders develop an intense emotional attachment to the items they have. Because of their anxiety, depression, guilt, and shame, hoarders frequently become isolated in their homes, and are unwilling to have anyone come into their space.

What Are the Symptoms of Hoarding?

Approximately one or two people in every one hundred have serious problems with hoarding. The signs can start as early as the teen years, but they get more intense with age. While the condition can get more problematic in older age, the disorder is well-established prior to that time. The symptoms typically include any or all of the following:

- An inability to discard possessions, often accompanied by an intense emotional attachment to the items in the home;
- Keeping or collecting large amounts of objects with little or no monetary value--for example, junk mail, newspapers, magazines, or items that the person intends to repair or reuse;
- Anxiety when attempting to clean or clear things out;
- Difficulty organizing or categorizing possessions;
- Indecisiveness regarding how to store things;
- Difficulty managing daily tasks like cooking, cleaning, or paying bills;
- General distress;
- Suspicion of anyone who touches your possessions;
- Poor or deteriorating relationships with family or friends;
- Obsessive thoughts and actions;
- Functional impairments;
- Clutter blindness.

Additionally, psychologists have identified some typical patterns seen with hoarding. Specifically, there are three identified patterns, referred to as hoarding life cycle patterns.

Hoarding Life Cycle Pattern #1

This pattern is identified by a person who can, in fact, regularly decide about discarding items, but develops a problem through the extreme acquisition of objects. In this case, the clutter can be brought under temporary control, but it will recur with the arrival of newly acquired items. In this pattern, there is an ebb and flow to the clutter that is dependent upon the number of items arriving versus those that are being discarded at any given point. The individual is able to give items away to people they know will appreciate the object, use it, and take good care of it. If this individual experiences some kind of destabilizing setback that upsets the checks and balances created by regularly discarding items, the clutter can significantly increase to levels where the individual feels overwhelmed. Such setbacks are ultimately inevitable.

Hoarding Life Cycle Pattern #2

This pattern is one where discarding items occurs infrequently, but so do acquisitions. Both occur at lower rates, and thus, the hoarding pattern takes longer to develop into a serious clutter problem. Still, the potential is there, and the situation will ultimately result in extreme clutter. This pattern is associated with object acquisition, rigid saving, and a focus on the possibility of using the item. These kinds of hoarders want to get the most value from the items they collect. They compare the price of the item with the use they get out of it. If they don't believe they have gotten their money's worth out of the item, they are unwilling to let it go. They equate keeping the item with somehow retaining the money they spent on it. Even if the item proves not to be as useful as they had anticipated, they still compare the money spent on the item's ideal value. Thus, keeping the item makes them feel as if they are getting their money out of it, even if it is only rarely used.

With this pattern, discarding items also happens differently. These hoarders will tell themselves that they are too busy to take the time to discard the item. They may, in fact, have genuinely busy lives, but though they tell themselves they will do it later, they never seem to find the time. They overcommit their time and energy in a way that they are overscheduled, which is but another symptom of compulsive behavior. Why are they keeping themselves so busy? This is an attempt to provide a justification for failing to face the problems their behavior is generating. They too are vulnerable to setbacks that can significantly and rapidly increase the clutter build up in their homes.

Hoarding Life Cycle Pattern #3

This pattern involves individuals who don't accumulate much more than the average person, but they never discard anything. Nothing that enters their home will ever leave it. They might have a recycling system, but somehow the items they collect never make into the recycle bin. They may also claim to be storing and saving items for others--a younger sibling's children, for example--but they never actually donate those items to the intended recipient. This offers the individual a noble cause as justification for their hoarding. It might take a while, but this will ultimately result in an extreme clutter situation. It's a particularly intractable pattern since the individual claims to be doing it for other people.

What Kinds of Things Do People Typically Hoard?

People can hoard many different types of things, but there are some common patterns with regard to what people most frequently tend to hoard. The following is a list of some of the more common items that people hoard:

- Newspapers and magazines;
- Books;
- Bills and receipts:
- Containers like plastic bags and cardboard boxes;

- Household supplies;
- Clothes;
- Leaflets and letters, including junk mail.

While these are the more common items that people hoard, there are other things as well. For example, hoarders might collect animals, which they frequently don't care for properly. Recent data also shows that some people hoard huge amounts of electronic data and emails that they don't want to delete.

Why is Hoarding Disorder a Problem?

There are several reasons hoarding is a problem. First, it can completely take over a person's life. Their excessive clutter can become so overwhelming that they can have trouble even getting around their house. It can affect their work performance, personal hygiene, and their relationships. Hoarders often feel shame because of their disorder, and that frequently makes them reluctant or unable to have visitors. They don't even want to allow a repairman into their house for essential repairs. And, all of this can cause isolation and profound loneliness. Furthermore, the excessive clutter can pose a health risk to anyone living in or visiting the house. The clutter can make cleaning difficult, which in turn leads to unhygienic conditions that can result in rat or insect infestations. Moreover, the chaotic storage poses a fire risk and can block the exits. The clutter also makes it easy to trip and fall, and if the stacks of items are high enough, the clutter can even fall on anyone in the house, causing serious injuries. All of this adds up to a very serious problem.

What to Do If You Suspect Someone is Hoarding

It can be very distressing to watch someone you love succumb to this disorder. And, if they don't realize they have a problem, it can be very difficult to convince them to seek help. But, that's exactly what you should do. Be sensitive about the issue as you explain your concerns for their well-being. It's also important to reassure them that no one will be going into their homes and throwing anything away. Explain that therapy involves empowering them to conquer their disorder and a doctor can help explain the options for how to accomplish that. It's best to seek a referral to someone who is familiar with hoarding disorder and any associated conditions like OCD. Whatever you do, you don't want to call someone in to clean the clutter. That can cause more problems than it solves.

How are Hoarding Disorders Treated?

Treating a hoarding disorder is difficult even when the patient realizes they have a problem and wants to solve it. One of the main treatments is called cognitive-behavioral therapy or CBT. With this type of therapy, the therapist helps the person get at the root of their disorder. To truly conquer the problem, people affected with this condition have to understand the underlying psychological reasons for the behavior. It works by changing how the person thinks (cognitive) and acts (behavior). To do that, the therapist will explore how the patient thinks about themselves, the world, and other people. Moreover, the therapy helps the patient understand how they think about these things affects their thoughts and feelings.

While CBT therapy sessions occur over a long period of time, they are often also accompanied by "homework." They also frequently include sessions in the patient's home where the therapist will help them work on the clutter. It's important to be patient since the therapy typically lasts for months before the ultimate goal is achieved. And, the goal is not simply to declutter the home; the goal is to help the person overcome the psychological reasons behind the hoarding behavior and help them improve their decision-making and organizational skills.

It's also important to reassure the patient that a therapist won't throw anything away; rather, their goal is to help the person regain control over their own life, to identify and challenge any underlying beliefs that are behind the problem. As the patient is able to start discarding items in their home, they understand that nothing bad has happened and that they are becoming better at organizing the items in their home. With that for encouragement, they will have more motivation to continue working on the problem. By the time the patient has finished the treatment, they will have a much better understanding of their own behavior, and they will have a plan to avoid relapsing into more hoarding in the future. It is also possible that the therapist may elect to administer antidepressant medications. These include medicines called selective serotonin reuptake inhibitors (SSRIs). These medications prevent a buildup of serotonin on nerve receptor cells in the brain. A buildup of serotonin is associated with depression.

In sum, it's evident that this condition is far more complex than simply shoddy housekeeping. The effects of the disorder are serious and sometimes dangerous. If you're reading this book, you likely understand that either you're a hoarder or someone you love is. If, as a hoarder, you're not seeking treatment, the first step is to find a therapist with experience in treating hoarding disorder and seek help. It's an important part of getting to the root of the disorder. If you're already receiving treatment, then this book is a useful tool with decluttering tips you can use to support your treatment.

For anyone serious about changing their life, they have to treat this disorder like they would any other illness. They must seek professional help, and use other sources, such as this book, to help overcome the challenges that they encounter on the path to healthy living.

Chapter Summary

In this chapter, hoarding disorder has been defined and described. Specifically, the following topics have been covered:

- The definition of hoarding disorder;
- The signs of hoarding disorder--compulsive collection of items and chaotic organization;
- Associated conditions with hoarding disorder;
- How the individual views their clutter;
- The typical treatment for hoarding disorder;
- What to do if you suspect someone you know is a hoarder.

The next chapter will focus on recognizing how important ongoing support and therapy is for the treatment of hoarding disorder.

STEP 2: RECOGNIZING THE IMPORTANCE OF ONGOING HELP AND SUPPORT

Hoarding disorder can be a difficult condition to treat, because often, people don't really understand the negative impact of this problem on their health and their lives. For that reason, they frequently don't believe they need any kind of treatment. This is particularly true if the items or animals that the person hoards offer them psychological comfort. That makes it difficult for them to think about losing those items or animals, and if someone suggests they should get rid of them, they will often react emotionally, becoming very angry or expressing frustration.

Insight Problems

Many researchers believe part of the problem in recognizing the need for help is a lack of insight into the severity of their symptoms and the need for change. In fact, studies have shown that people with obsessive-compulsive disorder who hoard have worse insight into their own symptoms of hoarding than people with OCD who do not hoard (Owen, 2020). And, that lack of insight causes significant problems that include avoiding seeking help, withdrawing early from treatment, and/or failing to comply with the homework assignments given by the therapist. Moreover, it is this lack of insight that frustrates family members and friends, and can eventually drive them away. Frequently, the only way that people finally agree to seek treatment is after they have been threatened with some negative consequence like eviction or divorce. They may enter therapy to prevent the negative consequence rather than because they believe they need help. That is precisely why treatment is often ineffective.

Once they do accept that they need some kind of help, it is important for them and their family to realize that recovery from a condition as complicated as hoarding disorder doesn't occur overnight, and it is an ongoing process. It is something you deal with on a daily basis. For that reason, asking for help is imperative as part of the process of treating this condition. There are a number of therapeutic options, but the most common psychological therapeutic choice is cognitive-behavioral therapy (CBT).

Cognitive Behavioral Therapy

Cognitive-behavioral therapy has shown great promise for treating hoarding disorder. Research (International OCD Foundation, 2020) indicates that some 70 to 80 percent of individuals with hoarding disorder show significant improvement after nine to twelve months of treatment with CBT.

This type of therapy helps people affected with this disorder get at the root of their condition; in other words, it helps them get at the psychological reasons behind their compulsion. But, that's not all CBT does. It will also help teach a patient strategies for preventing further hoarding behavior and decluttering their home. Furthermore, it helps to reduce their anxiety as they declutter their home, and it helps with organization and decision-making. Additionally, it helps hoarders to identify and challenge those persistent thoughts and beliefs that they have regarding acquiring and saving various items. It also teaches them how to resist the urge to acquire more items. More specifically, the following topics are what patients undergoing CBT will learn about and experience:

- **How to process information:** Part of the problem is that they have difficulty making decisions regarding what kinds of possessions they need, what to keep, and how to organize what they do have. Thus, treatment focuses on generating and enhancing skills associated with sorting, organizing, and decision-making.
- **Emotional attachment to possessions:** Many hoarders have intense sentimental attachments to the items they hoard. They are very reluctant to even consider discarding them. For that reason, CBT therapists will use techniques such as cognitive restructuring and exposure therapy to help challenge those beliefs. This will help the patient to explore the truth about the objects and their value as well as the consequences associated with keeping or discarding them.

Cognitive restructuring involves learning to identify and dispute irrational thoughts as well as negative automatic thoughts through the use of techniques like guided questioning, recording, and disputation. Basically, hoarders learn to test their ideas for accuracy before simply accepting them as true. The idea is to replace those thoughts that generate anxiety with more rational, positive thoughts that help reduce anxiety.

- **Beliefs about possessions**: Hoarders have intense beliefs about their possessions that they must maintain control over them. They feel that they have a responsibility to see that the item doesn't go to waste. For that reason, CBT focuses on restructuring those beliefs by critically examining their validity.
- **Behavioral Avoidance**: One of the problems that hoarders have is in coping with situations that generate anxiety. That anxiety is what causes them to avoid having to deal with the situation, something they have been doing as the items have been piling up in their home. CBT teaches them how to not only face what feels initially like an overwhelming situation in a systematic manner, but also to develop different strategies for anxiety-producing situations. A CBT therapist will help the patient replace their avoidance with adaptive coping strategies that they can use throughout their life as difficult situations arise.

The therapy ideally involves regular home visits as well as visits to settings where clients are triggered in their hoarding behavior, for example, flea markets, yard sales, and shopping centers. Additionally, the therapy rotates its focus among the behaviors of acquiring items, sorting and organizing materials, and discarding unnecessary, redundant, or useless items. The progression of the therapy depends on individual circumstances--some find decluttering is the best first goal and tolerate the stress that brings while others find it easier to first get control over acquiring behaviors.

The progress made by patients being treated for hoarding disorder depends in part on the ability of the individual to change their thinking. The goal is to reduce the emotional distress associated with losing possessions. To help an individual change their thinking, clinicians may employ discussion and CBT methods. CBT therapy typically progresses in the following stages:

Assessment: This is the stage where the clinician will assess the specific symptoms including how they interfere with everyday life, the safety problems they might cause, and any physical or other mental health issues that might affect treatment.

Formulation of a Personal Model of Hoarding Behavior: At this point, a therapist will work with the patient to ensure they understand the causes of hoarding disorder and how their own symptoms have developed into a serious problem. They will explain the causal factors, such as psychological vulnerabilities, problems processing information, and the beliefs and emotions associated with the importance of objects. From there, the therapist and patient can begin the process of gaining insight into how these factors have contributed to excessive acquisition and saving that has resulted in the significant build-up of clutter.

Motivational Interviewing: These are techniques that help patients to consider how their hoarding behaviors fit within their own value system and the goals they have for their life. These will help to sustain a patient's motivation for change.

Excessive Acquisition Reduction: While patients may be initially directed to avoid situations where acquisition behaviors are triggered, the focus of this part of CBT is to gradually expose the individual to those situations that act as triggers for their hoarding behaviors. Examples include driving to a store, but not going in, then going in, but not touching anything, and then picking up items, but not buying them. This kind of practice can help the patient develop strategies to resist the urge to acquire more objects and then they can progress to more challenging situations.

Skills Training: Hoarders typically have difficulty processing information, and that leads to significant skill deficits. They might, for example, have difficulty staying focused on tasks, have problems organizing items into logical categories, or have little ability to plan ahead to achieve their goals or solve basic problems. This kind of training will help them to develop those important skills, which will give them a healthy foundation for resisting hoarding urges.

Practicing Letting Go: This gives the individual the skills they need to part with their possessions. Typically, they will be encouraged to work from easier to harder items and make decisions about which to keep and which to let go. This is part of exposure therapy and it provides them with an opportunity to learn tolerance for the negative emotions that arise and to challenge those negative feelings to better understand and deal with them.

Therapy for Hoarding Beliefs: Throughout the treatment process, patients are encouraged to be mindful of their thoughts and feelings about acquiring and discarding possessions. This part of the therapy will help them explore those dysfunctional beliefs regarding the future usefulness of objects, concerns they have about waste, sentimental attachments, and the need to keep their memories alive. Therapists work with their patients to help them develop questions regarding the possessions in order to better evaluate the accuracy of their thinking. There are a number of methods that therapists use to help patients challenge their beliefs and consider alternative behaviors as they come to understand those beliefs are not realistic.

Relapse Prevention: As patients make progress with their hoarding behaviors, it is important that they develop good habits to replace the hoarding habits. Clinicians work with their patients in this regard. The good habits include things like putting things away immediately after they are brought into the home, cleaning up immediately after a meal or other activity, removing trash and recycling on a regular basis, and addressing those particularly difficult situations that vary between individuals. Therapists work with their patients to ensure they have developed good habits to meet the challenges that will surely arise in the months after treatment comes to an end.

In cases where anxiety is undermining progress, it is also possible that a therapist might prescribe medication. The medications frequently used for hoarding disorder include antidepressants like venlafaxine and paroxetine, but it is imperative that medication be given in conjunction with CBT. These types of medications are known as selective serotonin reuptake inhibitors (SSRIs). Serotonin is a neurochemical that is known to be associated with depression. As neurons--nerve cells in the brain--communicate with one another, neurochemicals like serotonin facilitate that process by bridging the gap between the nerve cells. The gap is called a synapse and serotonin crosses the gap and lands on a receptor cell on the other side of the synapse. There it accumulates until it is recycled. Normally, the brain takes care of this without help, but if there is any problem with that process, it can result in too much serotonin accumulation or too little. And, that can cause problems like depression or anxiety. Thus, if they're suffering from depression or anxiety, a CBT therapist might decide to prescribe one of these medications.

Supportive Relationships

As part of the healing process, it is vital to include family and friends, and CBT can sometimes involve family/relationship therapy. The support of family is critical to helping a hoarder as they confront difficult emotions and thoughts and learn how to change those negative patterns into productive, positive behaviors. The family's support can help inspire the afflicted person to continue making progress in their treatment and to persevere on the journey to healthy behaviors. For children with hoarding disorder, the parents are an important element in their treatment. In fact, parents often have to learn how to change their behaviors since they likely contributed to the problem in a process often called, "family accommodation." It's easy for them to think they are helping to alleviate their child's anxiety by allowing them to acquire and save the items they hoard. In fact, the opposite is true as the hoarding serves to increase anxiety. That's why it's important for the entire family to be engaged in the treatment process.

Ongoing Treatment

It is important to recognize that hoarding disorder is a very challenging issue. It is difficult to treat and recovery can take a long time. The ongoing support and therapy a hoarder receives from a professional cognitive behavioral therapy counselor as well as the support of family and friends are crucial for helping them persevere in the decluttering process. It's important to recognize when you make progress in this fight. Even small steps should be applauded, but it's also important to recognize that the treatment for hoarding disorder is an ongoing process that requires continued support to work through the significant problems associated with this disorder.

Chapter Summary

This chapter has covered the importance of seeking help and continuing supportive therapy throughout the decluttering process and beyond. Specifically, the following topics were covered:

- The difficulty with treating hoarding disorder;
- The insight problems most hoarders experience;
- Cognitive Behavioral Therapy (CBT) and how it can help;
- The adaptive coping strategies hoarders learn with CBT;
- The importance of supportive relationships.

The next chapter will discuss how to take control by setting goals and planning.

STEP 3: TAKE CONTROL THROUGH GOAL-SETTING AND PLANNING

It's important at this stage to discuss a little about goal setting and planning in general. There are a few simple things to remember no matter what the ultimate goal is, but this is also particularly relevant for decluttering in response to a hoarding disorder. It's important to be systematic when approaching the problem. Take it one step at a time and it will be far easier to achieve the desired goals.

Tip #1: Identify the Problem

It is important to understand the nature of the problem. It's a good start to answer the following questions:

- How is the clutter affecting their life?
- How will their life change when the home is decluttered?
- How do they feel about the clutter?
- How will they feel with the clutter gone?
- Do they avoid having people over because of the clutter?

- Will they have more of a social life when the clutter is gone?
- Is the clutter affecting their relationships?
- Will their relationships improve when the clutter is gone?

By answering these questions, the individual can identify the specific problem and the positive benefits that will result once the problem is resolved. It's good to have a clear understanding of the problem and write that down in order to see it in black and white. That will also help for tracking progress.

Tip #2: Define the Ultimate Goal

Ideally, this will involve more than simply cleaning or decluttering the home. It should also involve goals in other areas of life, like improvements in relationships or the ability to be more social. In a sense, this involves describing in detail what success looks like. For example, this might sound like, "When I have decluttered my home, I will happily invite people over for social events, I will feel like I live in a clean and safe environment, and I will have a beautifully organized home." It's important to be as specific as possible so that when the goal has been achieved, it will look as envisioned. Also, by stating specific goals, it's helpful for staying motivated and on course.

Tip #3: Create a Vision Board

The next important thing to do before actually starting with the decluttering process is to create a vision board that visually displays the reasons for decluttering. These are taken from the ultimate goals described in Tip #2. It's helpful to visually represent those goals, and that includes more than simply a clean, well-organized home. That should be on the board too, but so should how it will *feel* to have a decluttered home. For example, a vision board for this process could contain happy pictures of oneself as well as family and friends. It's also a good idea to include pictures of tidy shelves and cupboards as well as pictures that represent being able to easily find things. Posting inspirational quotes on the vision board is also helpful for motivation. And, when there are moments of doubt or when the anxiety levels rise too high, examining the vision board can help to calm an individual and get them back on track.

To create a vision board, the following items are required:

- Some kind of board--it could be a cork board or poster board, although it might be more helpful to have a board where it's possible to pin items to and move them around.
- Scissors, tape, pins, or glue to affix pictures to the board.
- Magazines from which images and quotes can be cut.
- Photographs of happy family and friends.
- Time--most people need about an hour or two to put together a vision board. It should be a stress-free activity since this will be a source of inspiration and motivation. Therefore, it's important to make sure to allow for enough time to get it just right.

The vision board is something that they will look to regularly for inspiration, so it should be placed in a prominent location in the home where it can be seen easily.

Tip #4: Make a Map of the Home

Now that the long-term, general goals have been identified, it's time to examine the home and break down the declutter process into a series of short-term, specific goals. This begins by making a map of the home. Each space in the home should be examined, and areas within each space should be identified for processing. This will be important for prioritizing areas for clearing the clutter.

Tip #5: Grade the Clutter

Once the map of the home has been made and the areas of focus identified, it is now time to grade the clutter. Use a scale of 1 - 3, with 1 being the least cluttered and 3 being the most cluttered. This will make it possible to identify the areas that will take the most work to clear, and that will help with prioritization when planning the work.

Tip #6: Plan the Work

It's critical that when planning the work, it be broken down into manageable goals. If not, the task will simply seem overwhelming and there will be an urge to abandon the plan and relapse into hoarding. Remember the adage, "How do you eat an elephant? One bite at a time." By breaking the decluttering process down into a series of small, easily achievable goals, it will help to not only achieve those goals, but to stay inspired and motivated. Additionally, those small goals can be celebrated when they've been achieved.

As part of the planning process, the grades assigned to each space should be used to prioritize areas for addressing. It's also a good idea to identify spaces within each room for priority work. Start by identifying those short-term goals--areas for decluttering--that can be achieved within a short period of time. For example, perhaps you have identified a closet within the most cluttered room to clean first. That's something that may take a week to break down the clutter, but at the end of that week, that clean closet is something to celebrate. And, that builds much-needed motivation.

By identifying a series of small areas that represent short term goals, it's possible to build a plan for the work. Mark each area on the map of the home in order of priority. It's also a good idea as part of the plan to state how the goals will be accomplished. That will be discussed in more detail in a later chapter, but suffice it to say here that it's important to have a system in place that you can follow with the least amount of uncertainty regarding how to accomplish the goals. That's particularly important for a hoarder since the urge to give up is a frequent problem.

It's also a good idea to make note on the plan of longer-term goals. These can include things like decluttering an entire room, then an entire section of the home (for example, the upstairs), and finally, the decluttering of the entire house itself.

Tip #7: Write Everything Down

Writing everything down is a good way to ensure that you follow the plan. It's easy to get off-track if nothing is written down in black and white. In fact, there are a number of psychological benefits to writing everything down. They include the following:

- **Positive emotions:** Whether writing about stressors or goals, writing things down can create a happier, more positive attitude. For the person affected by this disorder, writing things down helps develop self-discipline for following the plan and decluttering each space, it helps with problem-solving when deciding what to do with the hoarded items, and it helps to alleviate anxiety. All of these benefits lead to more positive emotions.

- **Clarity**: When you have a written plan, it alleviates the stress of having to make decisions. The decision is made, and it's in the plan. The goals, priorities, and intentions behind the decluttering process are clear and easily accessible. That makes it easier to actually tackle the work.
- **Documentation**: Writing everything down helps document the process, the intent behind the work, and it helps keep track of the progress.
- **Sense of accomplishment**: By writing out the plan, it will be easier to document accomplishments. And, there will be something to mark off the list, which helps create a sense of satisfaction with a job well done.
- **Boosts efficiency**: Having a written plan eliminates the need to decide what to do on any given day. The plan has it all laid out. That helps to get going on the work quickly, and in that way, it boosts efficiency.

Tip #8: Set a Start Date

With a written plan and work priorities identified, it is important to set a start date. A plan is great, but if it never gets initiated, it doesn't do much good. By setting a date to start the work, it will create motivation even as it allows for necessary preparation. Subsequent chapters will discuss allotting a specific time frame for each task in your plan as well as the general start and end date for the work. This will help eliminate any procrastination as well.

With these 8 basic tips, it's possible to create a plan for action. It's important to remember a few things. First, be realistic about the difficulty in achieving each goal and the time it will take to do so. It's also important to involve other people in the process. They will help establish a sense of accountability as well as support and encouragement. They are, in effect, a source of motivation. And, they can help to alleviate the anxiety that may arise during the decluttering process.

Another important concept to include in any decluttering plan is a way and time to evaluate progress. Perhaps, it is done on a weekly basis whereby they would consult the map and see how many of the identified goals for the week were actually achieved. If all of them were achieved, that's something to celebrate, and it should be celebrated. For that, it's important to establish a system of rewards. Rewards might include going to dinner at a nice restaurant or a favorite activity. It's probably a good idea to avoid rewards that would require accumulating more objects. Instead, go someplace fun or do something fun, but in any case, be sure to reward those goals that have been successfully achieved. If some of the goals were not achieved, celebrate the ones that were and tweak the plan. Don't get discouraged and give up just because some goals were not met. Keep going and pretty soon, all of the goals will be achieved. By celebrating the accomplishments achieved, that will provide more motivation to keep going.

Chapter Summary

This chapter discussed how to take control of the declutter process through setting goals and planning. Specifically, the following topics were discussed:

- Being systematic in the approach to setting goals and planning the work;
- Identifying the problem and describing success;

- Creating a vision board for inspiration;
- Making a map of the home and prioritizing the work;
- Planning the work, writing everything down, and setting a start date;
- Tracking progress and rewarding achievements.

The next chapter will present information on designing a schedule and managing time.

STEP 4: DESIGN A SCHEDULE AND MAKE FRIENDS WITH TIME

At this stage, they have created a plan for decluttering their home and identified a start date. The next step in the decluttering process is to create a schedule for the time frame for achieving each decluttering goal. This time frame should ideally include plenty of time for each task, and allow for taking it one small space at a time. It's also important to remember that sometimes a task will take longer than anticipated, so build a little cushion into the schedule. If a particular task takes even longer than the allotted time with the cushion, it's critical not to use that as a punishment or to think of it as failure. As long as they don't give up, they won't fail.

Begin with the Map

The map of the house with the identified prioritized areas will help to design a schedule for the decluttering process. Begin by choosing between one and three prioritized areas. Assign dates to each area for decluttering. Be sure to be reasonable about the time frame needed to declutter each room. Not doing so will set them up for failure and can be discouraging. It's also important to understand that it's unlikely that an entire room will be decluttered within one span of time. It's much better to break the room down into smaller spaces. For example, if the first space is a bedroom, that can be broken down into the following areas: closet, dresser drawers, bedside tables, and any other storage areas like a trunk at the end of the bed, or a storage container under the bed. Also, if things are piled on the floor, then be sure to include floor space, which can also be broken down into separate spaces, e.g., floor space to the right of the bed, floor space to the left of the bed, and floor space in front of the bed.

How much time is needed to declutter an entire space depends on several factors. These include whether you have the entire day to devote to the project, only a few hours in the evening after work, how much clutter is present, how large the space is, and whether or not difficult emotions arise that slow the progress. It's a good idea to allot more time than might be necessary for a space so as to avoid feelings of failure or discouragement. If there's a lot of clutter and only a few hours a day that can be devoted to the decluttering process, then a small space could take anywhere from one to three weeks. The amount of time it takes to fully declutter a space is not as important as consistent progress. For planning purposes, set a time frame that is much more than you think you'll need.

The Pomodoro Technique

More important than the overall time frame is the work time devoted to decluttering a single space. The Pomodoro Technique is a popular time management technique invented in the 1990s by Francesco Cirillo. The technique is named for the tomato-shaped timer Cirillo used to track his work as a student. It's a helpful technique for breaking down any large task or series of tasks into short, timed intervals that will help to boost efficiency. It also trains the brain to stay focused during those short intervals and it improves attention span and concentration skills. The technique is cyclical in that work is accomplished in short sprints followed by regular breaks. That helps ensure consistent productivity, and the breaks bolster motivation and creativity.

To demonstrate how the technique works, imagine the task is decluttering a table. To start, set a timer for 25 minutes and work on the decluttering until the timer rings. When the timer rings, take a 5 minute break before beginning a second 25-minute interval. This results in enhanced concentration during the work period, which in turn, reduces the overall time needed for the task. In that way, it helps dramatically improve efficiency. This technique can be applied to decluttering each space within each area of the house, and it will help to reduce the time it takes to entirely declutter the home.

The Two Minute Rule

This is another method for increasing productivity that was designed by consultant David Allen. It helps form new habits and complete tasks by breaking them down into small steps. Again, imagine the table to be decluttered--begin with some action that takes no more than two minutes. Perhaps, start by collecting papers into a pile or clearing away coffee mugs--either of those is something that can be completed within two minutes. Keep track of the time to ensure you're accomplishing these micro-goals within the two minute time period. This technique produces an enhanced sense of accomplishment because it's possible to achieve a goal within a very short period of time. That motivates them to keep going and it generates a long list of accomplishments in a very short period of time. That makes the overall goal of decluttering the entire home seem much more achievable. This rule will also help to prevent procrastination, because after all, the job only requires two minutes. And then, it seems much easier to take on another two minute job, and then another. Once one job is started, it's easier to keep going. That's how this method increases productivity.

Set Schedules for Each Task in Each Space

It's important not to try to do too much at once. By approaching the entire decluttering process one task at a time rather than thinking about the whole thing, it will help keep you focused on goal-oriented tasks. While it's important to set a schedule for each task, it's also important to be flexible. There are a number of things that can delay the process, which makes it difficult to judge the time required for each area or even each space within the areas. Some tasks will take longer than expected, and sometimes, challenging emotions and thoughts will arise during the process. It's important to address those as they arise since that is an important part of the healing process. Self-compassion is a crucial part of confronting those difficult emotions, and it's also acceptable to adjust the schedule as the need arises. The most important part of the decluttering process is to keep going, to make constant progress. The overall time frame is not something that is set in stone, but continuous progress is critical.

Chapter Summary

This chapter discussed the importance of setting a time frame for the decluttering process. Specifically, the following topics were covered:

- Using the map to assign time frames to each area of the house;
- The Pomodoro Technique for increasing efficiency by breaking down large tasks into smaller ones;
- The two minute rule to increase productivity by taking on tasks that take less than two minutes;
- Setting schedules for each task, but remaining flexible and practicing self-compassion.

The next chapter presents information on creating a system for decluttering.

STEP 5: CREATE A SORTING SYSTEM AND PREPARE YOUR RESOURCES

Being fully prepared is an important part of the decluttering process. It will help them feel organized and give them a system to follow so that when they begin, they won't be distracted by constant delays created by the need for more supplies.

Create an Organization System

Before it is possible to effectively declutter your home, it's important to devise an organization system. Decluttering will be difficult since there is likely a long history of finding it impossible to throw things away. By devising a plan, it will help to know what to do when faced with the clutter. A useful organization system is what's called the "Four Box Method." This method involves preparing four containers to use during the declutter process for each area of the house. They should be clearly labeled with "throw away," "donate/sell," "storage," and "put away." The creation of these boxes alone can generate anxious feelings, but they must remember that they are the one who is in control. If they struggle with the idea of throwing things away or donating or selling them, return to the vision board and remind them of exactly why they're doing this.

The Four Box Method

The four box method helps to keep the decluttering process moving along. It prevents the need to figure out what to do with the items that you're not keeping. As mentioned, the idea is to create four boxes for each area of the house to be decluttered:

- **Throw Away:** This box is for any item identified as unnecessary and not worth selling or donating. Donation centers often require that items be in good condition, and if an item's not in good enough condition to donate, it is probably also not in good enough condition to sell. That only leaves discarding it if it is not an item that you're keeping.
- **Donate/Sell:** This presents an opportunity to be generous and think about the uses someone else might have use for the item. If it is something that isn't really being used, then it's preferable to make it available to others who might find more uses for it. Additionally, it could provide them with a financial benefit if they're able to sell it.
- **Storage:** This box is for things that they can't part with but also don't need regularly. Because you'll be keeping these items, it's important to organize them well. That means making an inventory of the items in the box, and storing that inventory with the box or writing it on the outside. That way, should the need for an item in this box arise, it will be easy to find. It's also a good idea to group similar items together. For example, any items associated with the kitchen can

be grouped in the kitchen storage box or out of season clothing can be put in one box.
- **Put Away:** This should be the smallest category, and it should contain only those items that will be out on a regular basis. A good way to check for that is to first determine a place where each item will go. If there is something that doesn't have a place, that might indicate it belongs in another box. If they end up with too many of these items, to avoid cluttering your home again, then it will be necessary to reassess their importance. Revisit the vision board to remember all of the goals for the project and the reasons behind those goals.

Once the four box system is in place, it is then possible to declutter according to category. Begin with items that have little sentimental value and that are clearly trash. From there, it is possible to move on to the category of items that are identified as no longer useful, but that aren't rubbish. These are for donations or to sell. Then, move on to the materials to store and those that you will keep. Just because they've moved on to a different category doesn't mean there won't be more items for that box. But, by decluttering the area by category, it is possible to eliminate the majority of items in the space that belong in that box. And, it will be possible to organize the materials in a space at a higher level. For example, begin with trash versus not trash, then donate/sell versus keep, and finally, store versus use regularly. In this way, the process of decluttering will be much more efficient. Finally, be sure to make an inventory of the contents of each box. It might be a wise idea to buy labels for this purpose.

Gather Supplies

Once the organizational system is ready, it's time to get

resources in the form of cleaning supplies. Here's a list of some of the supplies necessary for cleaning and decluttering:

- Heavy-duty trash bags;
- Empty boxes;
- A mop;
- A bucket;
- Disinfectant spray;
- Cleaning cloths;
- A dustpan;
- A broom;
- A vacuum cleaner;
- A step ladder;
- A shovel, particularly if the home is extremely cluttered.

It's important to be aware that simply gathering supplies might trigger hoarding behavior, and that can result in an excess of materials. That will just add to the problem, so it might be a good idea to enlist the help of family and friends to get these supplies. Provide them with a list of supplies, and they can make sure to get just what is needed and no more. That will prevent triggering hoarding behavior while buying supplies.

It's also likely that the decluttering process will result in an enormous amount of rubbish to be discarded. It might be a good idea to arrange for a skip/dumpster bin to be delivered to the front of the house. That will help ensure that once rubbish is identified, it can be discarded immediately before there is time to rethink the decision. It will also prevent simply moving the items to a different part of the house where they become part of a separate clutter pile.

By creating an organizational system, such as the four box

method, it will be much easier to declutter any space. It will also reduce the amount of thought process involved in deciding what to do with an item. Gathering supplies will help in the preparation so that there will be no reason to delay decluttering any more. At this point, they have a plan, a time frame, and an organizational system for decluttering their home. It's time to get to work!

Chapter Summary

This chapter presented information about a good organizational system, the four box method, as well as the materials needed for decluttering any space. Specifically, the following topics were covered:

- The four box method;
- What goes in each of the four boxes--trash, donate/sell, storage, and put away;
- The supplies needed for decluttering;
- What to do to avoid hoarding behavior while gathering supplies;
- Disposing of rubbish immediately by using a skip/dumpster bin.

The next chapter will present information on decluttering one small area at a time.

STEP 6: TACKLE ONE SMALL AREA AT A TIME

Once a plan is in place and the supplies have been gathered, it's time to begin the decluttering work. If the job is big and help is required, be sure to have a family member or friend on hand for help and support, or hire an assistant for the day. It might also be a good idea to make lunch before beginning so that taking a break is easier to do. When it's time to get to work, here is how to proceed:

Start with the Map

Begin with a small area on the map. It should be a high priority area, but it's best to begin in an area with minimal items that have sentimental value. The bathroom is a good choice to tackle first. It's less likely to have items of sentimental value and it's an area that's regularly used, so when it's clean, it will engender a sense of achievement every time it's used. Beginning with areas of low sentimental value is helpful until the person has acclimated to the process. Once the process is well-established, it will be easier to tackle those areas that will cause more challenging emotions to arise. When the area on the map is identified, choose a small space within the area to begin. Remember to use the two-minute rule and the Pomodoro Technique as you proceed.

Select a Space within the Map Area

Once the area is selected, choose a space within the area to begin the actual decluttering process. For example, if they select the bathroom to begin, start with the cabinets under the sink. Another small space in the bathroom would be the medicine cabinet. These small areas will be easier to declutter, thereby providing a sense of accomplishment as that small goal is successfully achieved.

Stage the Belongings

Before they begin the actual work of staging, set a timer to work for 25 minutes of uninterrupted work--the Pomodoro Technique. Within that 25 minute time period, divide the tasks into two-minute jobs. For example, one two-minute job in the medicine cabinet might be removing and dividing the expired medication from the current medication.

Once the timer is set and the two-minute jobs identified, begin working by staging the belongings. That means remove them from where they are stored or piled to an area where it's possible to see them clearly. This can add a shock value to the process. Hoarders are often not aware of just how much stuff they've accumulated. This technique is also useful for revealing duplicates of items. Once the items are staged, it's easier to identify what is trash, what can be donated or sold, and what needs to be put away or stored.

When staging the belongings, they can be divided into categories if there are different types of items. For example, if the space is that medicine cabinet in the bathroom, perhaps there are current medications, expired medications, makeup materials, dental floss, and band-aids in the cabinet. Separate the items by type to better identify what and how many of each are present. As already mentioned for this example, one way to divide medications is by expiration date--those which are expired versus those which are current.

Declutter by Category

Now that everything is staged, it will be easier to see what and how many items are present. This will make it easier to further divide the items into the four box categories of trash, donate/sell, store, or put away. Begin by removing the items in the trash category. Once the trash box is full, take it out to the skip/dumpster bin and empty it immediately. If this presents a problem for the individual, have the family or friend assisting them do this or accompany them to the dumpster. Then, move on to the donate/sell category and put those items in their box. Place the storage items in their box and begin the inventory of storage items. Finally, place those items that will be kept where they belong after thoroughly cleaning the area.

Clean the area thoroughly before moving on to the next space. Each time a task is completed, like cleaning out that medicine cabinet, be sure to appreciate the success. It's crucial during this stage to monitor for distress. It's quite likely that any hoarder will experience challenging emotions as the decluttering proceeds. It's important to acknowledge those feelings and practice the CBT techniques for understanding and dealing with them. Having a support network on hand, particularly in the beginning of the declutter process and when clearing areas with numerous items of sentimental value. To be effective in support through this process, it's important that family and friends agree to a support schedule when they can be present to help as the individual proceeds through the declutter process. If the distress is severe, it is also acceptable to hire a professional cleaning service rather than decluttering personally. The point is to clear the clutter and treat the behavior that resulted in the accumulation in the first place.

It's common at the beginning of the process for them to feel overwhelmed by the amount of clutter. Don't let that become discouraging--remind them of that old adage about how to eat an elephant; one bite at a time. Visit the vision board to remember all the reasons for doing this work. The images of clean spaces and happy family events in a clutter-free environment serve as potent reminders for how life can be once the job is done. It's also important to call on the support network as needed. Hoarders will typically alternate between feelings of shame and hopelessness until real progress can be seen, and therefore, it's essential to have supportive family, friends, and even therapists at the ready to assist as necessary.

Finish the Area Before Moving On

Completely finish the work in the target area before moving on to another area. Again, it's important to consistently check in with the types of feelings and thoughts the person is experiencing as they proceed with decluttering. The negative feelings that arise should be thoughtfully considered and dealt with in accordance with the CBT techniques learned in therapy sessions. It's important to acknowledge positive feelings that arise, too. As areas are decluttered, it's common to feel a sense of satisfaction and accomplishment. These feelings should be savored and used for further motivation. And, the success of clearing a space should be celebrated, too. Remember that it's a step toward a healthier, happier life.

Review Accomplishments

Once an area has been cleaned, it should be checked off on the map. That engenders an enormous sense of satisfaction, which then provides motivation for continuing the process. It should become apparent through the decluttering process whether the individual is ready to handle the feelings they're experiencing during the process. If it is generating too much distress as they are attempting to throw things away, there are options to consider that can help. Family, friends, or a professional cleaning service can take over when the affected individual doesn't think they can continue. They should not interpret this as a failure; in fact, if they are having someone else continue the declutter process, that is still a success. Their main job is to manage the negative emotions and thoughts that are arising as they move on with decluttering their environment. That is the real work of treating this condition. A decluttered environment is merely a side effect of the healing process.

Chapter Summary

This chapter has presented information on how to proceed with the decluttering process. Specifically, information on the following topics has been covered:

- Selecting a high priority, low sentimental value area to begin;
- Selecting a small space within the area;
- Using the pomodoro technique and the two-minute rule;
- Staging the belongings;

- Decluttering by category;
- Finishing one area before moving on;
- Reviewing accomplishments and progress.

The next chapter will present information on how to handle deciding what to do with specific items.

STEP 7: ERASE THE MAYBE - ASK YOURSELF QUESTIONS

It's so easy for anyone to vacillate when trying to throw something away. For a hoarder, it's even harder. That's why it's important to know the individual's style or personality and to take it one individual object at a time, asking some very specific questions about what to do with it. Which box to put it in? Additionally, it's a good idea to set strict guidelines that determine what to do depending on the answers to those questions. The following tips can make the process much easier.

Hoarder Personality

There are different kinds of hoarders, and it's helpful to know the style of the clutter accumulation. That will be helpful for identifying weak spots and clutter areas that might be particularly problematic. Most people fall into one of three categories:

- **The Disorganized Collector**: This person buys duplicate items because they don't have an organized system for storing them, and then, when they need

the item in a hurry, they can't find it. For that reason, they end up buying another one and the cycle starts anew.
- **The Saver**: This is the person who worries that they might need the object in the future. They save it, "just in case," but rarely actually need the item. They typically feel this way about every object regardless of the likelihood they actually will need it.
- **The Chronically Overwhelmed**: This individual feels constantly overwhelmed, and since they don't know where to begin with the declutter process, they consistently give up trying. As they accumulate objects, they may consider clearing them out, but the job feels like it's just too much, so they never do.

Be Prepared

Just like it's important to tackle one space at a time within the house, it's also important to make decisions about one object at a time. But, it's also critical to be prepared for those justifications that will undoubtedly arise. For example, many hoarders will use one of the following phrases in accordance with the personality types above. The phrases are: 1) "I have to go through those," common for the chronically overwhelmed, 2) "But, I need it," or a common saver variant, "Someone could use that," and 3) "I need a new one of these," common for the disorganized collector. It's helpful to actually write these phrases (or whatever common justification phrase the individual uses) down. That way it's possible to anticipate the objections that might come up during the decluttering process.

When these phrases do come up, it's important to challenge them, so the person can see how they're a symptom of dysfunction. For example, "I have to go through those," can be challenged with, "That's what we're doing now." "I need it," or, "I need a new one of these," can be challenged with, "When was the last time you used it?" If the individual can't remember or knows it's been more than a year, then they really don't need it and they certainly don't need a new one.

Ask Questions

For each object, it's a good idea to ask some specific questions about the item. They include the following:

- When was the last time this item was used?
- How important is this item?
- Does it have a specific use?
- If the answer is yes, what is that use and how often is it used?
- Did the person even remember that they had this item?
- Is this the only one of these the individual has?
- Is it so important that they would trade a sense of inner peace for it?

These questions will help you narrow down the decision about what to do with the item. For example, if it isn't something that gets used regularly or that the person even remembered having, then it probably isn't a necessary item to keep. That should help bolster the decision to throw it away or donate it to charity.

Set the Rules

It's a good idea to set specific guidelines regarding what to do depending on the answers to those questions. If these guidelines are set up and all parties agree to abide by them, then the decision is pretty much made depending on the answer to the questions. The questions and their answers can be set up like a flowchart. It could look something like this:

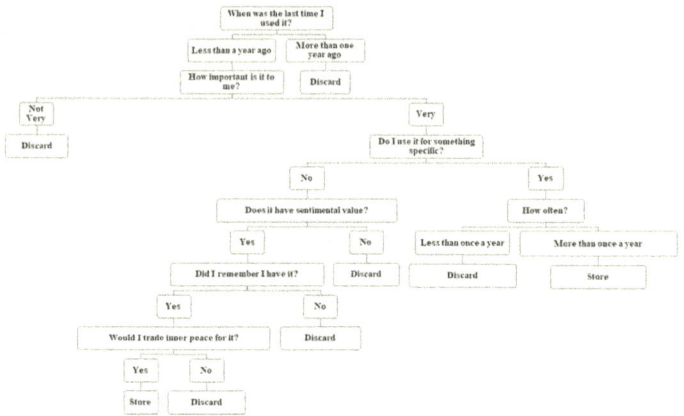

The answers to the questions on the flowchart leave little room for guesswork. The individual simply answers the questions and follows the flow. That will help eliminate any vacillation. If it's necessary to justify the decisions further, here are a few lines of logic that can help give the process more structure:

- If it hasn't been used in the last year, throw it away or donate it. Realistically speaking, if the object hasn't been used in that time, it's not something that is needed. There may be certain exceptions--for example, it's possible that a jack for the car hasn't been used in the last year, but that kind of item should be kept--but, generally speaking, this is a good guideline.
- If it is not something that the person even remembered having, then it can't have much sentimental value and it isn't very necessary--throw

it away or donate it. Truly sentimental items are something that most people will display somewhere in the home and remember having.
- If it is something that is sentimental, it's important to consider if it's worth a sense of peace to keep. A memento from a vacation taken years ago might have sentimental value, but particularly if it hasn't been on display, it's probably not something worth sacrificing a sense of inner peace. Take a picture of it so that it can be stored digitally and throw it away or donate it.

To determine whether it is something that should or can be donated, it's helpful to ask a series of different questions:

- Is it in good condition?
- Is it in good enough condition to sell?
- Who is it designed for?
- Can it help someone else?

Most charities require that donations be in an acceptable condition, so if it isn't, then it goes into the trash box. It's possible to see how these questions form part of a system for determining what to do with the objects in your house. By setting down specific rules for what to do depending upon the answers to the questions, it removes the guesswork and leaves less room for indecision that can stall the process. This produces a specific plan of attack that streamlines the decluttering process. But, there's another rule that can help at this stage.

Use the OHIO Rule

The OHIO rule is used to help determine whether fears about letting go of an object are rational. OHIO stands for Only Handle It Once. Once the answer to the questions asked above yields a definitive action, and the object has been placed in the appropriate box, it should never be handled again. Of course, those items put in the "put away" box will be handled again when they are put away, but they should be put away as quickly as possible to ensure that there really is a place for them, and then, they can be enjoyed. For the rest of the boxes, leave those items alone, and move on to the next object.

This process can create anxiety in a hoarder. If the distress is significant, ask "What is the worst that can happen if the item is discarded? It's a good idea to allow them to express the fears they have about discarding the item. It's also important to validate those fears and show them compassion. No matter how unlikely the fears are, to an individual afflicted with hoarding disorder, they are real and imminent. By allowing them to express their fears, it is then possible to use CBT exercises to challenge those thoughts and emotions. That helps the individual to work through and challenge their own negative thoughts and fears, which then gives them the power and control over their response to decluttering. This makes them stronger as the process progresses.

It is important to constantly check in as the decluttering progresses. The individual should be encouraged to voice any and all distress so that it can be properly dealt with, and the internal healing can proceed. They should not be teased or judged for their feelings, because their feelings are valid. They need to voice them to be able to challenge them. And, they should know that should it get too stressful, it's always an option to call in help from family and friends or a CBT therapist. This will help keep the decluttering process on track, and more importantly, it will help them begin to get control over their worst fears.

Chapter Summary

This chapter has presented information on taking as much of the guesswork out of the decluttering process as possible. These specific topics were covered:

- Hoarder personality types: the disorganized collector, the saver, and the chronically overwhelmed;
- Preparation for typical justifications for each hoarder personality;
- Questions to ask about each object to determine which box it goes into;
- The OHIO rule;
- Constantly checking in with the affected person and how they are feeling.

The next chapter will present information for when the individual is unsure what to do with an object.

STEP 8: HAVE A SOLID STRATEGY FOR WHEN YOU'RE NOT SURE

For most hoarders, an excuse to delay a decision presents a risk for abandoning the declutter process. For that reason, it's best to have a plan of attack for those times when a person simply doesn't know what to do with an object. There will certainly be those types of objects, and thus, to avoid problems, a solid strategy will help. The following tips can help in such situations.

Create an "Unsure" Box

Creating an "unsure" box can be useful for those items they're not certain about. This is, however, a strategy that should be used with care. It's easy for a hoarder to want to put everything in that box. One strategy to avoid that is to only allow one unsure box for each space. That way, the box can't be used too frequently. It's also a good strategy to employ the flow chart for these types of items. If the object hasn't been used in more than a year or if the person didn't remember they had it, then that makes a strong argument for discarding or donating it.

If an unsure box is created, then it's important to also make a specific plan to revisit the box within a certain period of time, for example, six months. If, when the person later revisits that box, they have forgotten what was in it, or if the items in it were not needed in that period of time, again, it's a good argument for discarding the objects therein. If, on the other hand, the individual uses one or more of the objects in that box on a regular basis or finds a place in the home to display the item(s), then there is the answer.

It's also possible to get an answer more quickly. Maybe sleeping on it will help. Sometimes a period of unconsciousness can help with the decision-making process. Researchers have discovered that the brain is always working, even when a person is unconscious. During unconscious thought, the biases that a person feels during the waking state disappear. Thus, it's possible to weigh the importance of the components that are relevant to the decision more equally. That's why sleeping on it can be a helpful strategy. But, if this strategy is used, it's also important to resolve to make a decision in the morning.

The important thing, in this case, is to have a plan in place for dealing with those items. If the items are just put away in some box, the problem has not been resolved, and the box becomes another hoarded object. This is another situation where it's important to have a plan that all parties are willing to follow. It's fine to take more time to make a decision by thinking about it for six months, but it's important to follow through on it. If, in that time, there hasn't been a need for the object or it hasn't been missed, then that is essentially a decision made in and of itself.

Duplicates

Most hoarders have duplicates of many items, and so, this is another situation that requires preparation and a strategy for resolution. Often duplicates are of items that are commonplace and easy to replace, for example, kitchen spatulas. Even so, hoarders are typically fearful of losing their things or being left without something they vitally need. For most hoarders, they struggle with the fear of decision-making and heightened emotional reactivity as part of the compulsive desire to keep the things they have, and when they are faced with discarding items, they respond with intense emotional reactions. That's part of why it's difficult to convince them of the irrational nature of their behavior. Even if they know on an intellectual level that they can easily replace that spatula, the problem is the intense emotions they may be feeling at the thought of discarding even a duplicate item.

This is why it is important to understand how to respond to those intense emotions when they arise. Because hoarders commonly fall into what are called "thinking traps," it can be useful to know how to deal with these. These thinking traps can goad anyone into more compulsive behavior as well as cause them to delay or abandon their efforts to heal their disorder. That's why it's worthwhile to examine some of the common thinking traps experienced by hoarders and methods for challenging those thoughts. The following table presents some common thinking traps and examples of thoughts experienced by people with hoarding disorder.

THINKING TRAPS: EXAMPLES

Thinking Traps	Examples
Fortune-telling: This is where the person will make often catastrophic predictions about what will happen as they move through the healing process. These kinds of thoughts are frequently triggered by the decluttering process.	*"I know I'll mess this up."* *"If I throw this away, I'll need it and won't be able to find another like it."* *"I will never be able to overcome my anxiety."*
Black-and-white thinking: This is where the person will think about a situation in terms of extremes. It's either all good or all bad, a success or a failure. While the declutter process is ongoing, if it's not been completed successfully, it's common for them to consider it an utter failure. This is true as well when they are faced with decision-making around items they're unsure about. They can easily view that as failure. In reality, there is a lot of gray area between the extremes.	*"Anything less than perfect is a failure."* *"Why do I still have problems with this? I should be cured by now."* *"I can't decide what to do with this item--I have totally failed to overcome this disorder!"*
Mind-reading: This frequently occurs as the person is certain they know what family, friends, and the therapist are thinking about them and their condition. Their sense of shame spurs this trap on, since they believe everyone is thinking the worst of them. The problem here is that most of the individual's friends and family just want to help.	*"Others think I'm stupid."* *"She or he doesn't like me."* *"They all think I'm crazy."*

Over-generalization: The best way to recognize this is when the words "always" and "never" are used. This type of thinking fails to take all situations or events into account. Surely, everyone makes mistakes, but that doesn't mean they can't achieve their goals.	*"I always make mistakes."* *"I'll never be able to keep from hoarding."* *"I'll never get this house decluttered."*
Labeling: This kind of behavior is reflective of the negative thoughts that are common to people affected by this disorder. CBT has specific ways to handle these types of thoughts, and that's one reason it is critical to the treatment of hoarding disorder. These negative thoughts undermine self-confidence and self-esteem. It's imperative for the individual to develop strategies for neutralizing negative thinking.	*"I'm stupid."* *"I'm crazy."* *"I'm a loser."*
Overestimation or Catastrophization: This kind of thinking is the result of the anxiety produced by the negative and obsessive thoughts. The person typically envisions the worst-case scenario, often resulting in an extreme or illogical conclusion.	*"I will lose everything."* *"If I give up my stuff, I will never be able to have these things again."* *"I will be unable to function."*

A great way to help a hoarder overcome these kinds of thinking traps is to challenge those thoughts as they arise. It's important to clear this with the person's therapist, but by actively attempting to transform negative thoughts into positive ones, the individual will learn to deal with these kinds of thoughts as they arise. That's a skill that's useful for more than hoarding disorder. The following steps can be used to help reorient the thinking patterns.

- What was the situation that triggered the thoughts? Write this down and describe it in detail as it happened.

- What was the obsessive behavior that was triggered? Describe what the person was feeling the urge to do.
- Rate the strength of the feelings or urges on a scale of 0 to 10 with 0 being weak and 10 being very strong.
- Hoarder's interpretation of the feelings or urges--describe this in detail.
- Balanced alternative interpretation--what is another more reasonable interpretation of the situation?
- Rate the individual's feelings about the balanced alternative interpretation on a scale of 0 to 10.

It might be helpful to illustrate these steps with an example. Considering the spatula example above, feelings of anxiety can easily be triggered when the person is prompted to consider discarding the duplicate items. When they recognize that they are feeling anxiety, it is a good exercise to have them stop and describe the situation that triggered those feelings. They might say something like, "As I was cleaning out my kitchen utensils, I encountered duplicate spatulas. I immediately began to feel anxiety upon thinking about discarding the duplicates. I had an immediate, strong urge to hide the items rather than discard them so that I would have them should I need them. I kept thinking that I might run out of spatulas and be unable to cook my food. The feeling was very strong. I would rate it an 8 out of 10. It caused me to freeze, and I found I could not continue the declutter process at that moment. My heart rate increased as did my breathing. That caused me to feel shame, because I'm not better yet. I thought I was getting better, but I still have such anxiety over something as stupid as a spatula."

Now, challenge those thoughts with these questions:

- Am I falling into a thinking trap, e.g. *catastrophizing* or *overestimating danger?*
- What is the evidence that what I'm thinking is true? What is the evidence that what I'm thinking is not true?
- Am I confusing a thought with a fact?
- What would I tell my best friend if he or she had the same thought?
- What would a friend tell me about this thought?
- Am I 100% sure that _____ will happen?
- Has it happened before, and if so, how many times?
- Is _____ so important that my future depends on it?
- What is the worst thing that could happen?
- If it did happen, what would I do to cope with it, what strategies am I learning that could help me to handle it?
- Am I basing my judgment of this situation on my feelings or on facts?
- Am I confusing "possibility" with "certainty"? It may be possible, but is it likely?

With these questions answered, it's now important for the person to devise a balanced alternative interpretation of the situation. The first thing to do is identify the thinking trap. There are several kinds here--there are elements of black and white thinking, over-generalization, and fortune-telling. Identifying the specific thinking trap can help with the reorientation of the thoughts and feelings the individual is experiencing. So, what would be a balanced alternative interpretation? It could look something like this: "It's so easy to accumulate numerous items like these spatulas. They are inexpensive and easy to find. My feelings of anxiety about these duplicates are understandable given my disorder, but

I'm making progress by working to declutter my home. I understand that this is a process and it takes time. I resolve to be patient and compassionate with myself. Discarding duplicates is part of that process, and the urges the thought of that triggered are merely side effects of the healing process. I know that should I require another spatula for any reason, I can easily acquire one, and even if my current spatula broke while I was using it, I could still use other utensils to finish cooking my food. The anxiety that was triggered initially is completely understandable given the decluttering process I am undertaking. I will continue to declutter my environment, because I know I am strong enough to take control over my obsessive urges. I love a challenge and I can do this!"

The balanced alternative interpretation is compassionate and recognizes the difficulty faced by the individual when undertaking decluttering procedures. It's important for them to recognize the feelings that arise as they move through the process. That is part of the healing they are seeking. Helping them to see the alternative thinking processes that are available will help alleviate their stress, and it will also train their brain to think more positively. Like any other habit, negative or positive thinking patterns create and strengthen neural pathways in the brain, which makes it easier for the brain to go down the same route the next time. For most hoarders, the negative thinking pathways have been strengthened over time. But, it's possible to retrain the brain to use strong positive thinking neural pathways instead. To do that requires vigilance with one's thoughts and feelings, and it requires taking the time consistently to replace negative thoughts with positive ones (Firestone, 2018; Oppong, 2018).

By dealing with negative feelings that arise during the decluttering process, it will also help to appreciate the strategies developed to deal with situations like duplicates and items the person is unsure about. That will help to keep the process going and everyone motivated.

Chapter Summary

This chapter has presented information on dealing with items an individual is uncertain about and duplicate items. Specifically, the following topics were covered:

- The "unsure" box and how to handle it;
- Why sleeping on it can help with the decision-making process;
- Putting the unsure box away for six months and revisiting those items at that time;
- How to deal with duplicate items;
- How duplicate items and uncertainty can cause a person to fall into thinking traps;
- The different kinds of thinking traps;
- How to challenge the validity of thinking traps and negative thinking.

The next chapter will present information on scaling down collections.

STEP 9: SCALE DOWN YOUR COLLECTIONS

Large collections of items can cause significant clutter, and often, they are things that don't really add to a person's quality of life. Still, people often spend many years collecting items in which they are particularly interested. Getting rid of those collections can be very distressing, so an alternate strategy is to scale them down instead. There are a number of ways to downsize any type of collection or memorabilia. It is important to understand that collections don't refer to duplicate items; rather, these are the kinds of things, like Hummel figurines, that form part of a collection. It also includes family memorabilia. While there are several reasons to keep these, they can add up to significant clutter, and that means it is necessary to develop a strategy for dealing with them. The strategy depends in part on the items being collected. The following strategies can be helpful.

Keep Some Items

Keep a few items from each collection instead of the whole collection. Pick out some of the more valuable or rare items in the collection. If numerous parts are kept in the home, keep them together so that they aren't scattered in different areas of the home. If the collection really is something of value to the person, then they should wish to display it. If not, it might be wise to consider if it is worth keeping at all. If the entire collection is something valuable, but it can't all be displayed, then one option is to display the more interesting or valuable items and store the rest. As with anything else that is stored, it's important to have an inventory on the box so that the items can be located easily. This will reduce the clutter, but make it easy to find the remaining items whenever necessary.

Consider Alternative Storage Strategies

Keeping part of the collection can help to reduce the anxiety generated by thinking about getting rid of it, but it's also important to spend some time thinking about whether it really adds value to life. If the collection involves something like magazines, cards, or pictures, the question is whether these will ever be used. Furthermore, are they being stored properly? If it is something that the individual really wants to keep, it might be worthwhile to explore alternative storage strategies. Pictures or cards could be put into a scrapbook for storage. That would help provide them with proper storage where they could be protected from deterioration due to environmental exposure. This would also provide them with a way to easily access the collection and show it to family and friends. For other types of items, like magazines, it might be worthwhile to consider the value of keeping these kinds of items. For this kind of thing, it might be better to keep some of the collection--the most notable or important issues, for example--and donate the remainder to a library where they can properly curate the collection. It might even be possible that they will make a note of the name of the individual who donated the collection.

Family Memorabilia

Collections also include family memorabilia, and that can be particularly difficult to downsize because of the attached sentimental value. These kinds of materials are also often tied to family histories and a sense of heritage. Many hoarders attach a sense of responsibility in overseeing the family heritage. That can make these kinds of things particularly difficult to deal with during the decluttering process. So, how can these kinds of items be dealt with when decluttering? It can be helpful to answer the following questions:

- **Do I love this and/or will I use this in my home?** Though the memorabilia that many people inherit from their family may be interesting, the items are often not something that they will really use in their home. They frequently start out keeping them because of feelings of obligation, but the reality is that unless the item is something that is being used, why store it simply for reasons of family history? The family history can be documented in other ways. For example, it's possible to photograph the item and describe what is known about its history and the importance to the family--for example, when was it acquired, is there a date associated with it, or is there a particular relative who originally bought or made it. Documenting that kind of information adds value to the item. Then, if it is not something being used, it can be donated or sold along with its provenance or history. Antique dealers will want that kind of information. And, the person still has the information about the item and its place in their family history.
- **Is this item really valuable to the family history?**

There are a number of things that people acquire over the course of their lifetime. No one knows that better than a hoarder, but many of those items are not particularly significant in the life of the owner. Much of what a person might inherit will be nothing more than useless items that have little value to their family history. These might include things like paperwork that has no value or items that, though old, were and are still commonplace, meaning they will have little value as antiques. Those kinds of things can easily be discarded.

- **Is this something my children will want someday?** There are certain things that children may eventually appreciate having as they grow older. War medals, family artwork, or items made by family members are possible examples. These are the kinds of things that might be worth storing to give to children someday. But, it's also true that many things won't hold the same sentimental value for the children as they might for older generations. Grandma's china might be important to her daughter, but her granddaughter might find it outdated. Thus, those things that are unlikely to hold meaning for the younger generations can be discarded.
- **Are the items in good condition?** This is an important consideration for whether to keep them or discard them. Old books, photographs, and other memorabilia might have real value, but if they aren't in good condition, that can negatively impact any resale value, and if it is not possible to properly curate them to prevent further deterioration, there is no reason to keep them. It might be worthwhile to find someone who can try to salvage those kinds of items and either donate or sell them to that person.

- **Is there something unique about the item?** Another consideration when deciding whether to keep or discard an item is if it is, in some way, unique. Antiques that have real value are usually rare. Items that were mass-produced or for which there are numerous examples will have less value than those items that are unique. If there is a question, it might be worthwhile to take the item to an expert who can help to evaluate its value. If it has no value, then it might be better to discard it.
- **If I do not want to display the item, do I have space to store it properly?** This is another important consideration. If the item will not be on display, is it possible to store it properly so that it doesn't deteriorate? If this is the decision, it's also wise to ask what purpose storing it will serve. Why keep something that won't be used or displayed? If the individual feels significant distress at making a decision regarding the item, perhaps for reasons of sentimental value, this might be an option, but like the "unsure" box, it is a good idea to revisit this decision in six months.

Letting go can be a difficult process, but it doesn't represent a loss, it represents a new beginning. It's helpful to remember the reasons for decluttering, and to focus on the new, positive feelings that will result from a decluttered environment. If the person is experiencing significant stress over this process, it might be time to revisit the vision board for reminders of just why this is a good process and all of the positive things to come.

Chapter Summary

This chapter has presented information on scaling down collections. Specifically, the following topics were covered:

- How collections differ from duplicate items;
- Strategies for dealing with collections;
- Keep some of the collection;
- Alternative storage strategies;
- How to deal with family memorabilia.

The next chapter will present information on how to be ruthless in the decluttering process.

STEP 10: BE RUTHLESS AND START AGAIN

When decluttering a house, it can be necessary to be absolutely ruthless. Having a plan in place to deal with the clutter will help with this. It can be difficult to do, but it's easier if it is done with much thought. That can be done for the kinds of things that are obviously trash. It's so easy to hoard household items, for example; things like beauty products, cleaning products, or stationery. The easiest strategy for trying to declutter their house is to just throw these kinds of items away. If necessary, make the decision to buy one replacement of every essential, but get rid of the old items. These are the half-filled shampoo bottles, the dozens of travel-sized soaps, and the hotel body lotions collected over numerous vacations.

Throw Them Out

As was mentioned, it's best to stage the items in a space that's being cleaned. For example, pull everything out of the cabinets under the bathroom sink, and divide the materials into piles by types. For example, put all of the cleaning supplies in one pile, things like toilet paper in another, and body lotion in yet another. With this strategy items that are trash will become readily apparent. Throw those things out right away without even thinking about it. Unless the item is something that is currently being used, it's best to get rid of it. That makes it easier to clean quickly, which results in a great sense of satisfaction. It also has the added benefit of helping to retrain the brain with positive feelings of a job well done. Remember that these kinds of items can be easily replaced, and so, don't allow anxiety about throwing them away to creep in and disrupt the flow of the work.

This is a good strategy for all items that don't hold sentimental value. It's the "fresh start" approach and it can help to clean things very quickly and easily. It is necessary, however, to be absolutely ruthless and rigidly consistent. In fact, it's best to act before there is even time to think about it--just scoop up all of those half-filled bottles into a trash bag, each and every one. Remember, this is an opportunity for a fresh start. By acting quickly and decisively, it will eliminate any question about what to do with the items. They're out before there's even a question about it. And, remember the OHIO rule. Once they're in the trash, they shouldn't be handled again.

It's common as part of this direct, abrupt activity to have some doubts, but these tips can help to alleviate any stress that arises as part of this process.

- **The 80/20 rule**: This rule was originally developed in relation to clothing. It states that a person generally only wears approximately 20 percent of the clothing they own an astonishing 80 percent of the time. While it was developed for clothing, it also works for other items. For example, most people tend to listen to 20 percent of their music collection 80 percent of the time. They play 20 percent of their video game collection 80 percent of the time, and so on. The goal for decluttering is to get rid of the things that go unused 80 percent of the time.

- **Don't worry about sunk costs**: Economists define sunk costs as those costs that have already been incurred and cannot be recovered. Except for rare items that increase in value over time, the majority of things in anyone's house can be thought of as sunk costs. The money it took to purchase them cannot be recouped. For that reason, it is better to think about the value added by discarding the item as part of the decluttering process rather than the money it cost to purchase it. That money is already gone and cannot be retrieved. Understanding the concept of sunk costs can help for making more rational decisions about the objects in the house.
- **If it's broken, don't fix it**: It's not uncommon to discover long-forgotten treasures as part of the decluttering process. But, if the item doesn't work, it won't help to keep it stored in the house for another moment, day, week, or month. Get rid of it. It's a sunk cost and it doesn't work. The decision is really an easy one, it's out.
- **Track the items that get used**: A clever way to do this during the preparation for decluttering is to put an item back where it lives to face the opposite direction of the other items around it. For example, if it's an item of clothing, hang it in the opposite direction of the other clothing items in the closet or put it back in the drawer upside down in comparison

to the other clothes. This is an easy way to see what is getting used and what isn't. When it comes time to declutter, it's easier to simply pull out those items that are not being used and discard them without thinking about it. Again, be ruthless.

- **Clear off flat surfaces**: Flat surfaces are easy places to pile things up, and they're a good place to start with decluttering. Be ruthless in throwing out the junk mail that gets stashed on the kitchen countertop, put away the pens used for making the grocery list in a drawer, and commit to keeping only a few essential, small appliances on those countertops. If there are items that never get used, consider donating them or throwing them out. Again, if it's something that hasn't been used in over a year, it's not important and can be discarded.

- **Store like with like**: Organize the storage for the items that will be kept so that like items are stored together. This makes it much easier to find them when they are needed, and it keeps everything organized nicely. This will not only help declutter the home, it will also reduce the stress of not being able to find something when it's needed.

- **Ask if an item will be used**: If there is something that can be used, that does not mean it is something that will be used. Be honest about the items that will be used, and donate, sell, or throw out those items that won't get used, no matter how interesting or useful they might be. If they won't be used, they're just taking up space.

- **More is not better**: It's not necessary to have two microwave ovens, four spatulas, or three blow dryers. It's easy to think that there's a back up if one breaks, but the reality is that most of these items are easily replaced if that happens. There's no reason to keep duplicate items. Be ruthless and get rid of them.

- **Avoid overthinking**: This is the benefit of acting ruthlessly and quickly, it's possible to avoid overthinking. If not, it's easy to get into a cycle of going through a complicated decision-making process. This can be avoided by having a strict policy regarding categorizing items and acting on the answers to the questions discussed in earlier chapters.
- **Don't judge**: As part of this process, problems will crop up and it's not uncommon for hoarders to judge themselves as inadequate. They've made the decision to declutter and seek treatment, but it can seem like a very slow process. And, when mistakes happen, they often feel discouraged. The job doesn't have to be perfect; it's okay to make mistakes, so don't judge too harshly. Treatment for hoarding disorder can be a long process and there may be setbacks. The important thing is to stay on track.
- **Have courage**: Beating this disorder can be scary. The person affected will confront some very uncomfortable feelings and thoughts during the decluttering process, and it takes courage to face those fears. The very fact that they have chosen to work through this process is a testament to their strength. But, it takes courage to face those fears and risk making a wrong decision.
- **Be patient**: Recovering from a hoarding disorder is a process. It will take time, so focus on those small victories, take time to celebrate the progress, and keep going.
- **Keep on trucking**: It's easy to become overwhelmed by the decluttering process, but it's vital to keep

going. Don't stop, even for a day. Maybe it's not possible to do more than just five minutes of decluttering a day, but that's good enough. It keeps the ball rolling so that the process is not stalled.

- **Be strict**: Make a commitment to the process by setting rules. For example, no TV until after the day's decluttering has been accomplished. This will help establish a reward for the day's efforts, and that can help in the process of retraining the brain, which is always looking for a reward.
- **Ask for help when it's needed**: There is never any shame in admitting that you require help. It's important to remember that it takes courage to ask someone for help. That might be friends or family members who are part of a support network or it could be a therapist. It makes no difference--reach out when necessary. Even if it just helps to have someone in the home as the decluttering process is proceeding, ask for help. Your support network is there for just this reason.

When setbacks are encountered, start the process over again. Don't let a relapse stop you from continuing with the healing process. Setbacks are inevitable when dealing with a challenging disorder such as this, but they don't mean that the process has failed. It's just a setback. Like every other part of the decluttering process, develop a strategy for dealing with setbacks. That may require calling the therapist or other members of the support network, but it also means reflecting on the reasons for the setback. It can help to keep a journal of the emotions triggered during the declutter process and any setbacks encountered along the way. Maintaining a journal can reveal patterns for the problems encountered during decluttering. For example, it might reveal the more common or powerful triggers, the patterns of thoughts and emotions that cause the greatest problems, and those emotions that come to the surface when significant progress is made.

Keeping a journal can also be a useful way to challenge negative thoughts and emotions. It can be used to document those thought traps and challenge their rationality. It can also help the person gain a deeper understanding of the underlying psychological problems that helped create the problem in the first place. This is a useful and illuminating strategy that helps with both the decluttering process and in maintaining a decluttered environment. And, it provides a non-judgemental outlet for the thoughts and emotions that so frequently grip a hoarder while attempting to declutter. This is where they can speak freely about the ideas that come to mind, the fears that threaten to derail their progress, and the hopes that keep them going. This is an area where a ruthless and strict attitude is necessary too. Be ruthless about recording those thoughts and emotions that arise each and every day. That's a good habit to develop.

Chapter Summary

This chapter has presented information on being ruthless during the declutter process. Specifically, the following topics were covered:

- Being ruthless in the process of discarding duplicate items;
- Tips for alleviating stress as part of the declutter process;
- The 80/20 rule and its broad application;
- If it's broken, get rid of it;
- Be patient and compassionate with yourself;

- Ask for help when needed;
- Respect the process.

The next chapter will present information on alternative ways to maintain cherished memories without adding to the clutter.

STEP 11: FIND AN ALTERNATIVE WAY TO KEEP MEMORIES

One of the biggest problems for hoarders are items of sentimental value. It's hard for anyone to let go of those, but it's also easy to attach sentimental value to an item as a justification for keeping it. That's why it's important to address these items in some very special ways. There are a few strategies that can help with these kinds of items.

Why is the Item Important?

Before undertaking this process, it is important to ascertain what the item really means to the individual. A few directed questions can help to understand the sentimental value it holds.

- Where did this item come from?
- What does it mean to the individual?
- Why exactly are they sentimental about it? Usually, it's not the object per se, but it's attachment to a particular person or event that gives it a sentimental value.

- Is this something that can be displayed in the home rather than stored?
- Is the item in good condition? If not, it's better to photograph it and discard the object.

Process Feelings of Attachment

It's also a good idea when processing sentimental items to process the feelings that they represent. It's important for people affected with hoarding disorder to understand that the object is not the feeling or the memory. Those are something that resides within each person. The object simply evokes the memory. Thus, it is possible to take a picture of the item and use that to honor those special people and events in each person's life.

Discarding items of sentimental value will take some time. It is difficult to let them go, and there certainly may be some objects the person will keep--perhaps the most favorite items or those in the best condition. It may take several sessions of decluttering to get through these kinds of items. That's okay, because it's important to process those feelings.

Get Rid of Any Guilt

Sometimes people hold on to items not because they are sentimental about them, but because they feel guilty. They might feel bad about a relationship with the person who is attached to the item, and they keep the item because they feel guilty about not repairing the relationships. Unfortunately, guilt is a useless emotion. It won't fix any relationship or undo any action taken in the past, and neither will keeping the item to which the sentimental value is attached. Guilt is a particularly unhelpful emotion that needs to be processed and let go of. Sometimes just recognizing the real reason behind the sentimentality can be enough to let go of the object, but other times it may be necessary to process the feelings in a different way. Here are a few tips:

- **Understand the feeling**: Before anything can be done about feelings of guilt, it is imperative to first understand the root cause. By identifying specifically what the individual feels guilty about, it will then be possible to move on from the feeling.
- **Talk about it**: As with almost any other feeling, it's important to talk it out with a trusted friend, loved one, or professional. They have a much less biased perspective on the situation and can offer the kind of support to help eliminate guilty feelings.
- **Practice self-compassion**: One way to do this is to imagine that it is a good friend who has this problem. It's helpful to think about the advice that a person would give to their best friend who came to them with this problem. Most people would be compassionate with their best friend, and if that's the case, why not be compassionate with themselves? This is not simply excusing bad behavior, but it is understanding the context in which the behavior occurs. The when and the why of the situation are important to understanding any reaction. By understanding those elements of the behavior, it is then also possible to have compassion for the response, even if it was inappropriate. Once there is self-compassion, it is possible to practice self-forgiveness, and that allows someone to make amends for their past actions. If they haven't forgiven themselves for their behavior, making amends will be more difficult.
- **Make amends**: Rather than living a lifetime with the guilt of past actions, why not simply make amends?

It's not possible to undo the action and it may not be possible to undo the consequences that ensued, but it is minimally possible to express remorse and ask forgiveness.
- **Ask a Pro**: If the feelings of guilt are too difficult to overcome, it's helpful to discuss them with a professional therapist. They can help the individual get to the root of their guilty feelings and move on from this distinctly unhelpful emotion.

Gifts Should Not Be Burdens

Many people hold onto items because they think the person will expect to see them when they visit. That may or may not be true, but even if it is, it's unfair for a gift-giver to have that expectation. It is, after all, a gift, which means it is the recipient's prerogative to do with it as they see fit. This can become a boundary-setting issue that might need to be addressed. If the gift giver were to ask about the gift, the recipient should be able to tell them that, though they appreciate the giver's thoughtfulness, the item just wasn't a fit for the home, and thus, it was given to someone who would truly appreciate it. It's important here to understand that no one controls another person's feelings, and if the giver is offended, they should also properly process their feelings to fully understand why. But, whether they do that or not isn't something under the control of the recipient.

Virtual Memories

One great way to maintain the sentimental value of an item without actually keeping the item is to create a digital filing system. This is where you take photographs of your sentimental items. By doing this, you can keep the memories the item represents without actually keeping the item itself. This is particularly helpful for things like childhood artwork, memorabilia, magazine articles, and any other kind of paper item. It's also great for physical photographs, letters, documents, and greeting cards.

A good way to start is by organizing a filing system on whatever form of Cloud storage is available--Dropbox, Google Drive, iCloud, Evernote, etc.. In these systems, it is possible to create folders for things like childhood memories, projects, arts and crafts, letters, important documents, etc.. Once that has been accomplished, it's a simple matter of taking photographs of the items. It might be a good idea, depending on the item to take a photograph of each side. Once the photographs have been taken, they should be uploaded to the cloud storage, and then the physical item can be discarded.

Uploading these items to their digital file immediately can help ease your anxiety around getting rid of the physical item. And, this can also be done for objects like ornaments or jewelry that you don't need anymore, but they remind you of someone special or a special event. The great thing about this technique is that it allows you to access your memories more easily than if you had to sift through piles of stuff in your house or even locate the item in a box somewhere. Additionally, knowing that you can see your treasured memories anytime you like can help ease your anxiety about discarding the item.

Donate Significant Objects

Another good idea for preserving objects that the individual feels deserve special respect is to donate the item. If it is an antique, it might be possible to donate it to an archive or local history museum. This is a great way to declutter without discarding the item, but the item should be researched in order to determine if it has value and will be accepted by the organization.

Pass It On

Again, for those objects which the individual feels have value, but which they don't wish to keep, a good option is to pass them on. Even though one person might consider the items trash, another family relative might find them valuable. Consult other family members to see if anyone would like to have the object or objects in question.

Repurpose It

For those items which are in poor condition or unfit for sale, it's always possible to repurpose the item into something that can be used. For example, the stone from a grandparent's ring can be reset in a band that's more modern. A board from an antique dresser can be turned into a floating shelf. That allows the person to keep part of the item for its sentimental value while getting rid of the remainder.

Keep Part of a Collection

Decluttering a collection with sentimental value can be particularly difficult. But, it is possible to keep part of the collection and let the rest go. For example, keep one or two items that are representative of the collection, person, or era and that will make it easier to let the remainder go.

Give It a New Home

Some items may hold a particular sentimental value, such that the individual has difficulty deciding between storing it forever and discarding it. For these kinds of objects, there may be another option. Perhaps, there's a friend who would love to have the item or someone else who really needs it.

That way, the individual can be assured the item is going to a good home.

Make a Scrapbook

Making a scrapbook is simple and requires very little in the way of supplies; it only requires a simple, unlined notebook and a glue stick. And, a scrapbook makes a good place to store documents or pictures that have sentimental value or are an important part of the individual's life. The items can be preserved without taking up too much space.

These are great tips for dealing with items of sentimental value or those memories that are particularly important to preserve. Memorabilia can be particularly difficult for individuals suffering from hoarding disorder to organize, store, or discard. It's tempting to want to keep everything that is part of an individual's life, but it is possible to keep the memories without keeping the items themselves. The most important part of the decluttering process, particularly when dealing with these kinds of items, is to process the feelings that will undoubtedly arise during this part of the process. Individuals with hoarding disorder should be encouraged to voice their feelings and helped as they attempt to process them. Once they have mastered that skill, the decluttering process will become much easier.

Chapter Summary

This chapter has presented information on how to deal with decluttering memorabilia and items of sentimental value. Specifically, the following topics were covered:

- Determining why the item is important;
- Processing any feelings that arise as part of the decluttering process;

- Getting rid of any guilt associated with a perceived need to retain objects;
- Preventing gifts from becoming burdens;
- Various options for dealing with memorabilia.

The next chapter will present information on organizing, labeling, and storing those items that will be kept.

STEP 12: CHANNEL YOUR NEED FOR CONTROL INTO LABELING AND ORGANIZING

Most hoarders have a compulsive need to control their environment; that's part of the hoarding disorder. But, the energy that's behind that can be put to a more useful purpose, like organizing the declutter plan and categorizing and organizing those items which will be kept. Part of the problem with clutter is the impact it has on an individual's physical and mental health. Aside from the environmental hazards created by clutter, such as dust, mold, and fire hazards, there are other effects on an individual's physical and mental health. Clutter affects food choices which can contribute to obesity. It also affects interpersonal relationships, and it contributes to stress and depression.

Benefits of Organization

There are a number of benefits to decluttering and getting organized. Organization can help individuals sleep better, it can reduce stress, improve relationships, and allow a person to focus on other areas of their life in order to free up time and energy for improvements in those areas. Organization can also reduce depression and anxiety, result in better food choices, and help an individual lose weight. Finally, organization can help an individual be more productive.

How to Get Organized

Once the individual's environment is decluttered, it's time to organize those items that will be kept and stored in the home. This is an important part of the process since the individual will be living with those items for the foreseeable future. As with the decluttering process, planning is key. It's essential to make sure there is a place for everything that will be kept. Then, it will be important to get the necessary supplies. Make sure that everything is ready prior to proceeding so that there is no reason to delay. It's also a good idea to proceed systematically as was done during the decluttering process. Use the map again and proceed through each area on the map. The plan is to clean each area well and put the items that belong in that space away. To do that, it will require some supplies, including containers and container organizers. The following tips should help with the process.

Tips for Getting and Staying Organized

Here are some tips to get the organization process going and to make it much easier to do:

- **Clean**: Before putting anything away, clean the areas where the items will go. It's important to make sure everything is clean to begin.
- **Buy storage containers**: It's important to wait until this point to buy the storage containers since they will be a source of temptation during the decluttering process.
- **Find a home**: For the items to keep, find a place for them. Be sure to find a place for every object. They

should be located in appropriate rooms of the house, and in appropriate spaces within the room. If there's any indecision as to where an object should go, don't just put it on an open surface. That makes it too easy to slip back into hoarding behaviors. Instead, create an unsure container, and when everything else is finished, then go back and make a decision about where to put the items in that box.

- **Categorize Containers**: Each container in a room where items will be stored should be categorized by the type of item they will contain. For example, silverware drawer, spare batteries drawer, etc. can all be categories for drawers. That makes it easy to decide what goes in that drawer, cupboard, or box. Labeling each container will provide an even greater sense of control over the individual's environment.
- **Use open containers**: Use open containers to initially organize items, and then place those open containers inside the appropriately labeled drawer, box, or cupboard. By using this kind of rigid system, it will help with resisting the urge to sink back into disorganized hoarding behavior patterns. It will also help when putting things away. It's easy to toss items into an open container.
- **Open spaces**: Don't clutter up open spaces like tabletops. To avoid this, it can help to place something like flowers on the table. That will help prevent using the open space as a dumping ground for other objects.
- **No stacking**: Don't stack objects on top of one another. It can be tempting to do just that, but that's a great way to create clutter. Make sure that everything has its own space without having to be set on top of something else.

- **Create spaces that have limits**: This will help to prevent acquiring excess items in any one category. For example, if one drawer is for utensils, then if that drawer is filled and there are still more utensils, that indicates there's more decluttering work to do. And, over time, as that drawer gets full, it will serve as an indicator that it's time to address the problem again before it gets out of hand.
- **Every container should have container organizers**: Within each container used for organization, it's essential to include container organizers. Rather than simply throwing items into a drawer, for example, use container organizers to separate the areas within the drawer for use in storing specific items. Rubber bands can go in one area and batteries in another. In this way, even the all-purpose drawer can be organized properly.
- **Eliminate clutter hot spots**: There are places in every home that seem to be clutter magnets. These include places like an entryway table, kitchen counters, and the dining room table. Clear these areas of clutter accumulation each night before going to bed. Making it part of the daily routine can help prevent clutter accumulation. It can also help to put something on tables, like a flower arrangement, in order to take up the space so that there is less available for clutter.
- **Store a discard bag in the closet**: Use this bag for those clothes that no longer fit, are stained or out of style, or that just seem unflattering. Everyone has likely experienced buying clothing that seemed to look good in the store, but when they get it home, it suddenly seems less attractive. This bag is for those

kinds of clothes. When the bag is full, it's time to make a donation to the thrift store.

- **Arrange items according to how frequently they're used**: Items that are used daily should be kept in plain sight or at eye level. Things used less frequently can be stored on higher shelving, and those things rarely used can be stored in an attic or storage shed. This will make it easier to find things that are used often, and it will also be easier to locate those things not used as frequently.
- **Be selective about what is brought into the home**: Be selective about what is brought into the home now that it's clean and organized. Consider what is needed, and for those things that are desirable, be sure they fit, there's space to store the item(s), and/or there are no unnecessary duplicates. It's also a good idea to use the one item in, one item out rule. If something is brought into the home, something should be taken out. That will help prevent unnecessary clutter buildup.
- **Set limits**: For those items like memorabilia or knick-knacks, assign them a limited area for storage. If that area gets full, that indicates there's no more room. Be strict about not bringing any more items in that category if the storage space is full.
- **Set a deadline**: For any unfinished storage projects, set a deadline. For example, by agreeing to host a family dinner, that will create a deadline for hanging those family photos in the living room. By making plans that will require the completion of the project, that will provide motivation to get it done.
- **Put things away**: Putting things away is a habit like any other, but it's a necessary one to develop in order to avoid accumulating more clutter. If things are not

returned to their proper location, it will be easy to accumulate significant amounts of clutter quickly. By putting things away after using them, it will prevent the clutter accumulation and take much less time to keep things clean. It will also make it much easier to find things when necessary.
- **Appraise the system**: Once a space has been decluttered and organized, take a look around to see if it looks clean. If it still looks messy, then there is more organization to be done. And, it can also indicate that improvements to the organizational system are necessary.
- **Be objective**: Look around the home in the same way a visitor would in order to assess any areas of clutter that can easily be overlooked. Walk through the home with fresh eyes and look for any areas of clutter build up. It can help to snap a picture of the room too. It can be easier to see clutter in a photograph that is easily overlooked when looking at the area.

By organizing and labeling spaces in your home, you'll regain a sense of control that your hoarding behavior had given you previously. Additionally, organizing helps your mental health by reducing anxiety and depression. The decluttering process will have been difficult, and you may find you have an increased anxiety level, but you can reduce that anxiety by taking back the control through organizing and labeling.

Chapter Summary

This chapter presented information on organizing belongings following the decluttering process. Specifically, the following topics were covered:

- The benefits of organization;
- How to get organized;
- Tips for getting and staying organized.

The next chapter will present information on a final, thorough cleaning.

STEP 13: A FINAL CLEAN

The final step in the decluttering process is to clean the whole area. Once everything is organized and put in its final place, cleaning will be an easier process. Each section will have been cleaned during the decluttering process, and thus, this part will not be as difficult as it would have been if it had been done sooner. At this point, deep cleaning will be the final step.

After years of hoarding, a deep clean will make sure the home is sanitary and a comfortable place to live. Here are a few suggestions for approaching a deep clean:

- Consider hiring a professional service, particularly for areas with heavy grime or in the event the task seems too daunting.
- If there are areas that need repair work as you're cleaning, fix these as they are encountered or hire a handyman to the job. This is important to ensure that the space is safe and in good working order.

That will also make it easier to resist returning to those old hoarding ways.
- Once the home is clean, remove any trash bags and take pictures of the home in its pristine condition. That will be a good reminder for all the reasons to undertake this process in the first place. It will also serve as motivation to stick to those future goals. The photos will also provide an easy reference for how nice the home looks when it is uncluttered and well-organized.

When undertaking the deep cleaning process, there are a number of things to consider. The first is that deep cleaning, like the decluttering and organizational processes, should be undertaken in a systematic manner. It's important to acquire all of the necessary supplies first, and then, proceed through the home in a systematic manner. The following information presents suggestions for how to proceed.

Supplies

As with any other part of this process, it's vital to have the proper supplies before getting started. At a minimum the following items will be required for a thorough cleaning:

- Disposable rags, scrub pads, or towels that can be thrown way when the job is complete;
- Two buckets--one for clean water and the other for dirty water;
- Degreaser, dish soap, and disinfectant spray--be sure to get enough of these for the entire job;
- Rubber gloves;
- An abrasive scrub pad;
- A spray bottle with a 1:1 vinegar to water solution. Vinegar is a great cleaner;

- A scrub brush and/or an old toothbrush;
- Cleaning products like glass cleaner, wood polish, etc.

For each of these items, be sure to get enough to finish the entire job. Obtaining the supplies prior to cleaning will be easier than having to stop and buy more supplies. Those kinds of delays can derail the motivation to keep going.

Deep Cleaning Process

As with the other parts of the decluttering process, this goes more smoothly if it is done in a systematic manner. Here are some suggestions for some of the more challenging areas of the home.

Deep Cleaning the Kitchen

Oven and Stovetop: The oven might have a self-cleaning feature, but these vary in how effective they are, and it's important to remove all materials that might be a fire hazard before employing the self-cleaner. Use the abrasive scrub pad and degreaser to remove baked-on food. An alternative to this is to make a vinegar and baking soda paste and let it sit on the food spills in the oven for about an hour before cleaning it off. Clean the baked-on food off the oven surface and then clean the wire racks.

Once the oven is complete, clean the stovetop by removing the pot grates and soaking them in hot, soapy water. If the oven is electric, it is also possible to remove/unplug the coils in order to facilitate the cleaning process. If the oven or cooktop has a slide-out tray beneath the burners, be sure to remove and clean those. Scrub all of the surfaces, including the control knobs, with a soapy sponge and a wet rag soaked in clean water. Be sure to also clean the hood fan and hood fan filter.

Microwave: Use a lemon and vinegar mix to loosen food splatters. Then, clean the inside with a soapy sponge and wet rag. Remove the plate platform and clean that using dish soap and water. Glass cleaner can be used to clean the microwave glass and keypad. Be sure to remove the microwave from its enclave and clean under and around it.

Toaster: Most toasters have a slide-out platform under the toasting chambers. Remove that and clean the crumbs. Clean the surfaces of the toaster with glass cleaner.

Refrigerator/Freezer: Defrost the freezer by unplugging the unit. When it has defrosted, sponges dipped in a baking soda solution are great cleaners for the interior. A little vanilla extract can be added to the mixture to give the entire refrigerator a nice smell. Don't forget to clean the drip pan as well as the rest of the interior. When the unit is clean, leave an open box of baking soda to control food odors. One box will last approximately two months. Clean the outer doors with a cloth dipped in mild detergent, or if they're stainless steel, use a commercial stainless steel spray. And, don't forget to clean the rubber gasket seals around the doors with warm, soapy water. At least twice a year, use a vacuum cleaner attachment with a long-handled brush to clean the condenser coils in the bottom grill or kick plate, but be sure to unplug the appliance when doing this. This will increase the efficiency of the refrigerator by 3 to 5 percent, and that can result in savings of $100 or more in electricity costs each year. Finally, clean out any old food at the same time as cleaning the rest of the unit.

Sink: The sink will likely become dirty from this cleaning process as well as normal use. Wipe it out with hot, soapy water. Be sure to pay particular attention to the crevices in the backsplash and around the faucet. Use a disinfectant spray to remove stubborn stains.

Dishwasher: Use a baking soda and vinegar mixture to clean the dishwasher. This will remove the soap residue build-up that accumulates over time. Use a cup of vinegar mixed with one-half cup of baking soda and run the dishwasher empty.

Deep Cleaning the Bathroom

The bathroom is another challenging area to clean, but it is a particularly important area to maintain in pristine condition. To clean it, focus on the following areas:

Grout: There are a number of grout cleaners that are available for cleaning the bathroom grout, but it's also possible to make a solution using one part bleach to 10 parts water. Fill a spray bottle with that mixture and spray it on the shower floor and tiled walls. Pay particular attention to any visible mold. Let the solution sit for at least 5 minutes before gently scrubbing the mixture off with a scrubbing sponge or an old toothbrush.

Shower Curtain: This is another area where mildew accumulates. If the shower curtain is washing machine safe, it can be washed that way. If not, or to clean the plastic curtain behind a linen curtain, use a bathroom cleaner. If the plastic curtain becomes too full of mildew, they are inexpensive and can be easily replaced.

Toothbrush Holder: This is easy to overlook and often gets very dirty. Soak the toothbrush holder in hot, soapy water to soften the residue. Use soap, a pipe cleaner, a straw cleaner, or any other fine brush to scrub the inside of the holder. Once the grime has been removed, run it through the dishwasher or put it in boiling water for at least 30 seconds. It can also be left submerged in vinegar for 30 minutes or soaked in a 1:10 bleach solution for 30 minutes.

Toilet: Believe it or not, this can be cleaned in three minutes. For the first minute, open the lid and squirt in some commercial toilet bowl cleaner inside the bowl and around the rim. Close the lid and spray an all-purpose cleaner or disinfectant on the outside of the bowl. For the second minute, grab some paper towels and wipe down the back of the toilet, handle, top of the lid, the inside of the lid, and around the base. Microfiber towels are also great for this purpose, and they're good for picking up lint and germs, but they'll have to be washed afterward. In minute three, open the lid and use the toilet brush to scrub the inside of the toilet bowl--don't forget the inside of the rim. Flush the toilet and rinse the toilet brush. To get the hinges of the toilet seat clean, use an old toothbrush to scrub around them.

Deep Cleaning the Rest of the Home

With two of the worst areas for cleaning--the kitchen and the bathroom--scrubbed clean, it's time to deep clean the remainder of the home. This involves the following tasks:

- Cabinets/Drawers: Empty these out and use the vacuum to clean out any debris. Then, wipe the inside with a clean, wet rag or a cleaning spray. Wipe down the cabinet faces as well.
- Doors: Wipe down the doors, doorknobs, and door frames for fingerprints and smudges.
- Garbage cans: Wipeout and sanitize the garbage cans, recycling bins, and wastebaskets throughout the house.
- Blinds: For metal blinds, remove them and take them outside. Lay them on the patio and dip a brush in

soapy water to scrub each side of the blinds. When clean, rinse them with a garden hose and dry them with a towel. Lay them in the sun to thoroughly dry them. Fabric blinds can be spot cleaned with an all-purpose cleaner using a rubber sponge. A vinegar solution also makes a good disinfectant cleaner.
- Faucets: Use vinegar to descale faucets and showerheads throughout the home, and be sure to clean out the aerators in the heads.
- Vent covers: Remove the HVAC vent covers throughout the home and wash them with warm, soapy water.
- Windows: Vacuum window sills and tracks, and remove cobwebs and bugs from the screens. Clean the windows with a window cleaner.
- Ceiling fans: Wipe down and clean the fan blades.
- Couch and Chairs: Remove the cushions, vacuum the creases, and move the couch to clean under and behind it.
- Carpet: Spot clean any stains on carpet and upholstery. There are a number of commercial upholstery cleaners available to use for this purpose.
- Dust and vacuum: Dust all surfaces including hard-to-reach ledges, windows, light fixtures, and the tops of cabinets and other fixtures. It's important to clean all of the places that are hard to get to during normal cleaning. As necessary, get out the stepladder to reach those high areas, but be careful not to fall.

Remember that if the cleaning process causes too much distress, there is no shame in hiring a professional cleaning service to do the deep cleaning. Many people who are not hoarders prefer to use professional cleaning services, and no one considers the fact that they do as a sign of failure. It's no different if a hoarder chooses to do the same. Just keep checking in with and processing any feelings that arise during the cleaning process. This is the final step in the decluttering process, and by this point, the goal of having a clean, organized home has been achieved. This is something to celebrate. Visit the vision board once again and post some pictures of the newly decluttered and clean home along with images of the happy faces of those who accomplished this goal. And, take the time to enjoy a reward, like a nice dinner or a fun activity.

Chapter Summary

This chapter presented information on the final deep cleaning once the decluttering process is complete. Specifically, the following topics were discussed:

- Suggestions for approaching a deep clean;
- The supplies needed;
- The deep cleaning process;
- Cleaning the kitchen;
- Cleaning the bathroom;
- Cleaning the remainder of the house.

The following chapter will present information on having a plan to stay on top of the clutter.

STEP 14: HAVE A PLAN FOR STAYING ON TOP OF THE CLUTTER

Once the home is decluttered and cleaned, it will be easier to maintain that cleanliness. To stay motivated to that end, it can help to keep those photos taken after the deep cleaning was finished handy as reminders of how nice the home looks when it's clean. That can also help to prevent a relapse into unhelpful, past hoarding behaviors. Now, the task becomes maintaining that level of cleanliness. As with the other stages in the decluttering process, it can be helpful to develop a system.

A system for cleaning consists of a routine that becomes habitual. Remember that creating a habit actually results in physical changes in the neural pathways of the brain. Once those pathways have been reinforced, the brain will actually create urges to engage in the habitual behavior. This is why it can be so difficult to overcome bad habits, but in this case, this mechanism is helpful for creating a good cleaning habit. To establish a habit, repetition is key, and one of the best ways to ensure repetitive cleaning behavior is to create a cleaning schedule.

Establish a Cleaning Schedule

People whose houses are always clean achieve those results by maintaining a systematic cleaning schedule. This can be divided into those tasks which are done daily, biweekly, and those which are done weekly. Then, there are also a few tasks that are done less frequently than that, but those go on the schedule too. The following is a sample schedule that can be adjusted for individual circumstances.

Daily focus and tasks: The daily focus is to keep dirt at bay. This type of cleaning will involve handling any messes that occur from normal living to prevent both dirt and clutter accumulation. This is something that helps keep everything tidy, but doesn't clean the more serious dirt. The tasks associated with daily cleaning are the following:

- Make the bed;
- Put any dirty clothes in the hamper;
- When there are enough clothes for a load of laundry, do it;
- Wipe the countertops after preparing meals;
- Wash dishes;
- Clean up clutter hot spots--these are the areas that seem to naturally accumulate clutter, like the entryway or kitchen countertops. By putting items away or discarding them daily from these areas, it will prevent significant clutter accumulation.
- Wipe out the kitchen and bathroom sinks.

Weekly focus and tasks: The focus here is a more thorough cleaning that focuses on those areas that don't require daily attention. Here are some tasks associated with weekly cleaning. These are spread throughout the week so that the task completed on any given day doesn't take much time:

- Sunday: Vacuum all carpets and rugs, and mop tile floors.
- Monday: Vacuum furniture.
- Tuesday: Wash bedsheets.
- Wednesday: Clean windows.
- Thursday: Clean bathroom.
- Friday: Clean stove.
- Saturday: Dust and wipe down surfaces to remove smudges.

Seasonal focus and tasks: The focus here is on deep cleaning. It doesn't have to be done very frequently, but when it is time, the focus is to remove grime from all areas that don't get much attention throughout the year. The entire house should be deep cleaned at least once a year, but it's also possible to divide that job into seasonal cleaning tasks. Here is an example.

- **Winter**: In December, clean out and wipe down all cabinets. When cleaning the medicine cabinet, dispose of unused or expired medications. In January, clean behind the refrigerator, washer, dryer, and all large furniture. In February, steam clean the carpets.
- **Spring**: In March, empty the closets and donate any unwanted or unused items. Re-organize the closet to prioritize clothes for the spring and summer seasons. In April, clean the window exteriors and screens. In May, wash blankets, comforter, duvets, and the remainder of any large bedding.
- **Summer**: In June, clean and organize the garage and/or basement. In July, empty, clean, and organize dresser drawers. Donate unwanted or unused items. In August, clean walls and retouch paint as necessary.

- **Fall**: In September, reorganize the closets and dressers for the upcoming colder seasons. In October, deep clean the refrigerator and freezer as well as the stove and oven. In November, consolidate and organize personal files.

By breaking up these deep cleaning tasks into monthly chores, it will make it much easier to follow through on the cleaning. Doing one task each month won't be as overwhelming as thinking about deep cleaning the entire house. There is room for flexibility, and of course, the schedule should be adjusted for individual circumstances, but once an appropriate schedule is in place, follow through on completing the tasks each month. Doing so will ensure the house stays clean and organized.

Here are a couple of other suggestions to maintain a clean, organized home.

Cleanliness Starts at the Door

Begin the process of keeping a clean, organized house at the front door. Leave shoes stored by the door and keep a pair of slippers to change into for wearing around the house. A mudroom entryway is a great help in keeping the house clean. That's where dirty shoes and outdoor clothing can be kept. That reduces the need to store those items in the main part of the house, and it prevents dirt from being tracked into the home interior.

A Place for Everything and Everything In Its Place

To keep an organized home, it's important to have a place to store everything down to the most minute detail. This includes things like keys, incoming mail (which should be sorted and disposed of as quickly as possible), and things like briefcases or other work-related items. Before bringing something new into the home, it is important to first ensure it has a proper place to be stored. If it doesn't, consider carefully whether it should be brought into the home.

One In, One Out Rule

This rule is just as it sounds--every time something is brought into the home, something else must be taken out. That helps to prevent duplicates and reduces the chance of building up significant amounts of clutter.

Stick to the Plan

Stick to the new organization system. Anything brought into the home should have a place to be stored, and it should fit in the individual system. If something is left on a free surface, it is important to stop and determine where it should go, and if, for that matter, it is something necessary to have. Complete daily and weekly tasks as scheduled.

Clean Frequently

It is important to keep the house clean to stay motivated to avoid clutter. This means cleaning frequently. In fact, for those areas that are used often, like the kitchen, it's important to clean them after every use. This is true for everyone, but it is particularly important for hoarders or someone living with a hoarder to be extra vigilant about this.

Miscellaneous Baskets

Create some miscellaneous baskets to collect objects throughout the day. Then, at the end of the day, return the items in those baskets to their permanent location. When relaxing, it's understandable not to want to put things away immediately, and that's where miscellaneous baskets can come in handy. Put items in the basket, and then before going to bed, take those items and return them to the proper storage area.

Filing Cabinet

A filing cabinet is a great item to have in the house in order to organize documents. This is where important documents can be easily organized and stored. When organizing the filing cabinets, label drawers in accordance with the types of documents that will be stored in each. For example, one drawer might be dedicated to financial documents while another is dedicated to titles and deeds. Still another might be dedicated to insurance documents. This will make it very easy to find these when necessary. A filing cabinet is not, however, a place to store junk mail. Be sure to get rid of that as soon as it comes in.

Impose Rules

Rules can ensure that the system will be followed. For example, one rule might be that there is no TV until the kitchen has been cleaned. Rules will help ensure that the home stays organized and there is little opportunity for clutter build up. By using rules to stay on top of the clutter, it won't get to a level that will be overwhelming.

Do It Now

Rather than putting a task off until a later time, it's a good practice to do it now. When it is evident that the task needs doing, completing it at that time will prevent a build of chores that need to be done. This doesn't work for every task, particularly those that need some planning or supplies, but for many things, like putting away that clutter, doing the task immediately can easily be done and that will help to prevent clutter build up.

Involve Family Members

Involving family members in the cleaning process can help make it go faster and in a much more enjoyable manner. One person should not be responsible for cleaning the entire house unless that person lives alone. If other people are living in the home, they should also have cleaning responsibilities. That helps keep everything clean and well-organized. Every family member should also be aware of the system and follow its guidelines.

Make Cleaning Fun

Cleaning and decluttering does not have to be a serious event. It can be fun. Turn on some mood music, light some candles, and dance around the room singing while cleaning. If kids are involved, turn the experience into a game with rewards for accomplishing the assigned tasks.

All of these tips can help turn cleaning chores into pleasant habits, and of course, they help prevent the build-up of clutter. With a plan to keep things clean and organized, the reward will be a beautiful, clean, and organized home that anyone would be proud to show off. That brings up one more suggestion--show off the clean, organized home. Make plans to host dinners or parties so that everyone can admire this clean, well-run home. That will provide both a reward for a job well-done as well as motivation to keep it clean.

Chapter Summary

This chapter presented information on having an organizational system for cleaning and decluttering regularly. Specifically, the following topics were covered:

- Establishing a cleaning schedule for daily, weekly, and monthly cleaning tasks:

- Organizational tips like the one in, one out rule and a place for everything and everything in its place;
- The importance of sticking to the plan and cleaning frequently;
- Imposing rules for cleaning and doing it now as well as making cleaning an enjoyable activity;
- Reward the accomplishment of a clean house by showing it off.

The next chapter will present information on continuing therapy for hoarding disorder and maintaining support networks.

STEP 15: CONTINUE YOUR THERAPY AND USE YOUR SUPPORT NETWORK

Therapy is a key part of the treatment for hoarding disorder. Even after the decluttering process has been successful, it is vital to continue with supportive therapy. While it is easy for hoarders to think they've conquered the problem, therapy can help prevent relapses, which are common. Part of the problem common to a hoarder is something called cognitive disorganization.

Cognitive Disorganization

Research (Weir, 2020) indicates that there is a parallel between the hoarder's disorganized home and a disorganization in cognitive functioning. People who suffer from hoarding disorder demonstrate deficits in sustained attention, working memory, organization, and problem-solving. Additionally, they exhibit lower visuospatial ability. An individual's visuospatial ability is their capacity to identify visual and spatial relationships between objects. This means that hoarders have difficulty perceiving or mentally representing where objects are located in space, and they are unable to manipulate that knowledge in their spatial working memory.

This negatively affects their ability to utilize that information to plan a sequence of movements.

These deficits in cognitive functioning are something reported by people with hoarding disorder frequently. They categorize it as difficulties with memory and being easily distracted. And, the degree of their own subjective impairment is correlated with their saving and acquiring behaviors (Weir, 2020). These cognitive problems appear to undermine the healthy reinforcement patterns that allow most people to let go of their possessions. For example, someone who doesn't cook much would have no problem giving up an unused griddle in their cupboard, but for someone with hoarding disorder, the griddle has a special meaning. The reinforcement pattern for the hoarder means that rather than associating the object with its usefulness, they attach special meaning to it, which makes it more difficult to discard. Attaching special meaning to objects isn't something that's unique to the hoarder, but hoarders are much more likely to apply sentimental meanings to almost every item then own. They are also much more likely to attach multiple meanings to each object. That further affects their ability to manage all of the associations they have with their possessions.

This cognitive disorganization displayed in people who suffer from hoarding disorder is visible with brain imaging technology. Scans using FMRI technology demonstrate that there is a lower connectivity evident in areas of a hoarder's brain associated with cognitive control. Moreover, there is greater connectivity in the default mode network, which is a brain network that becomes active as an individual's thoughts are focused inward as opposed to on the outside world. In comparisons of people with hoarding disorder, people with OCD, and healthy individuals in the process of making decisions about discarding their possessions, hoarders showed hyperactivity in the brain areas that compose what's called the salience network. This is the area of the brain that selects what stimuli are deserving of a person's attention. The same area of a hoarder's brain showed less activity than the other groups when considering other people's possessions. This indicates an overstimulation when it comes to considering discarding their own possessions, and it also suggests that those with hoarding disorder have difficulty making fine-grained decisions with regard to what is important. That's because their brain is always screaming that everything's important. Of course it would be difficult to discard any possession when this area of the brain is hyperactively insisting that everything is vital (Weir, 2020).

Treatment Options

This research serves to highlight the critical nature of continuous therapy to treat hoarding disorder. It will help the individual identify and address underlying psychological issues that tend to recur. With cognitive behavioral therapy, it is possible to identify and change the behavioral patterns that can lead to relapses, but that type of therapy takes time in order to treat the underlying causes of the behavior.

Cognitive Behavioral Therapy

CBT is by far the most successful method of treatment for hoarding disorder. There are a number of different applications of cognitive-behavioral therapy that can be useful in this regard. Some novel types of treatment include combining group cognitive behavioral therapy with online clinician support between therapy sessions. This method has shown promising results with higher group attendance and treatment gains that were maintained at the three-month follow-up assessment (Ivanov et al., 2018). Likewise, a blended therapy technique that involved twelve weeks of group therapy followed by eight weeks of online therapy showed promise in enhancing treatment effectiveness (Fitzpatrick et al., 2018). Other applications are specific to particular groups of hoarders. For example, a manualized CBT approach was used in a sample of geriatric patients with compulsive hoarding disorder. Though the results were limited in their efficacy, it highlights the need for innovative and population-specific treatments to this serious problem. The research indicates that problems with cognitive functioning are the underlying cause of hoarding disorder, and the higher frequency of cognitive impairment in this geriatric sample might explain the problems with this technique (Ayers et al., 2011).

The research into CBT for hoarding disorder indicates a significant decrease in symptoms with the best results obtained for discarding behaviors. But, despite positive results during the treatment process, most participants in the various studies on CBT treatments still showed significant hoarding behaviors after the treatment ended. This argues strongly for an ongoing treatment plan. While CBT is effective for reducing symptoms, it is not as effective as it is for other disorders like depression and anxiety. That indicates that CBT may not be the best option for every population. Younger people, for example, appear to benefit more from this treatment method than older people. That's a significant finding given that hoarding tends to get worse with age. For older adults, treatments modeled on interventions for individuals with traumatic brain injury may present a better option. In one study, participants showed a 40 percent reduction in symptoms with this kind of cognitive rehabilitation, and moreover, the improvements were maintained in a follow-up some six months after treatment (Weir, 2020).

While still far from a cure, those results are encouraging, and also speak to the need for ongoing therapy.

Motivational Interviewing (MI)

Another type of treatment technique that is often used in conjunction with CBT is motivational interviewing. This technique attempts to increase the motivation of an individual to make positive changes in their behavior. It does that by helping individuals connect values and goals with behaviors. The technique also makes use of brainstorming different ways to change those behaviors which are not in line with the individual's goals and values. MI has proved to be a successful adjunct therapy for treating individuals with obsessive-compulsive disorder (OCD). It is specifically helpful in getting patients to adhere to a treatment protocol.

MI first seeks to develop a positive relationship between the therapist and the patient in order to reduce patient defensiveness and increase motivation for change. It is a person-centered method that seeks to help patients explore the reasons behind their reticence or ambivalence to treatment. For people who suffer from hoarding disorder, limited insight is a common characteristic, and many hoarders, therefore, demonstrate a level of ambivalence about their behavior. They may recognize that their behavior is creating problems, but they simply cannot bear to part with their possessions. Thus, their overall goals are at odds with their thinking. MI has proven to be particularly helpful in assisting patients with maintaining their motivation as they are participating in non-acquiring and discarding exercises.

MI has two primary goals, the first of which is to increase the importance of changing the behavior. This refers to addressing the discrepancy between the individual's current living environment and how they would like to live. They have to experience that discrepancy in order to be motivated to change. MI creates the discrepancy for them to experience by exploring their life goals and values while at the same time realistically examining their actual experience in their cluttered home. Often they have pushed aside their basic values as the clutter overtook their life. Thus, MI discussions about what they actually value the most in life help set the stage for determining the value of their possession within the context of how they would really like to live their life.

The second goal of MI is to increase the individual's confidence that they can change. This goal requires some careful, dedicated work in evaluating the value of those possessions as well as in experimenting with different ways to use, care for, and discard objects. By helping patients discuss and make plans for change, MI can help them make significant progress with CBT in reducing their hoarding symptoms.

Skills Training

Skills training is another essential adjunctive therapy for hoarding disorder. It seeks to help hoarders learn how to organize their belongings within their home, how to use problem-solving techniques to deal with common problems that arise as they go through the declutter process, and how to make decisions about what items are necessary to keep and what items can be discarded. The cognitive disorganization common to hoarders is what causes problems with decision-making skills. Therefore, giving hoarders a specific skill set for making decisions related to their possessions is a valuable adjunct to cognitive behavioral therapy.

Medication

Certain medications have a treatment value for those who suffer from hoarding disorder. These medications typically seek to change the brain chemistry and assist in the treatment for hoarding by reducing the anxiety and depression frequently experienced in various stages of therapy.

Outlook for Hoarding Disorder Treatment

The most successful treatment options for hoarding disorder are those that result from early recognition and diagnosis of the problem. That increases the likelihood that someone affected by this disorder can successfully reduce the severity of their symptoms. If left untreated, hoarding disorder is quite likely to become chronic and to get worse over time. For that reason, people exhibiting signs of hoarding disorder should speak with their doctor or mental health professional as soon as possible. For those who know someone that they believe is affected by this disorder, they should consider contacting a mental health professional to find out how they can help that person seek treatment. It's a complex problem that requires compassionate solutions.

Ongoing Therapy

Most of the research into the effectiveness of various therapeutic options indicates that the symptoms can be successfully reduced. But, the research also suggests the need for ongoing therapeutic support to maintain that reduction in hoarding behaviors. It's also important for individuals who suffer from this condition to maintain their support system that includes their family and friends. As part of the reward for decluttering, the individual can now host family and friends in their clean, well-organized homes. That's a powerful motivation for maintaining a clean, decluttered environment. Thus, family and friends can help by accepting those invitations and marveling at the progress made by the individual in dealing with this difficult condition. Social connections are powerful motivators for change.

Still, decluttering is only part of the solution. It's also vital that sufferers of hoarding disorder are able to address the underlying psychological elements that are ultimately the cause behind their behaviors. A strong support system that includes family, friends, and ongoing therapy is crucial for maintaining a decluttered lifestyle where the individual can feel safe and in control. It's important to not only declutter the home, but the mind as well. That's why treating the psychological and emotional aspects of hoarding is imperative to true, long-term success in treatment. A clean, organized environment is, for the hoarder, a journey, not a destination.

Chapter Summary

This chapter presented information on the importance of ongoing therapy for the successful, long-term treatment of hoarding disorder. Specifically, the following topics were discussed:

- Cognitive disorganization and its role in hoarding disorder;
- Treatment options;
- Cognitive-behavioral therapy, its effectiveness and variations;
- The role of motivational interviewing techniques in the treatment of hoarding disorder;
- Skills training and the treatment of hoarding disorder;
- The outlook for hoarders and the importance of ongoing therapy.

The next chapter will present concluding remarks.

FINAL WORDS

For the 2 to 5 percent of US adults who suffer from hoarding disorder, keeping a clean, organized environment is a struggle. Because of the accumulation of clutter that often reaches dangerous levels, these individuals also suffer from intense feelings of shame and isolation. They don't have what most people consider to be a normal life. They live amidst the uncontrolled clutter that is representative of the cognitive disorganization that is also common among those who suffer from hoarding disorder. The need to acquire new possessions is obsessive in these individuals, and the intense emotional attachment they form with those possessions makes it extremely difficult to engage in a declutter process.

There is, however, help for this disorder, and no one who suffers from this should feel alone. There are millions of people worldwide who display symptoms of hoarding. The treatment of this disorder requires a solid plan of attack for helping those individuals suffering as hoarders regain a level of control over their own behaviors. It involves setting manageable goals and taking the declutter process one step at a time. During the process, it is imperative to be mindful of the intense emotions that frequently arise and threaten to derail any progress.

This book has described 15 steps to take to reduce the clutter that so seriously affects those who suffer as hoarders. These steps are proven to be effective, and by breaking the process down into one step at a time, they are relatively easy to do. Among the tools described to help them are the following:

- Making a plan for decluttering;
- How to assess each item and determine whether it should be discarded, donated, stored, or displayed in the home;
- How to store memories without keeping objects;
- How to process the feelings of shame, guilt, and anxiety that inevitably arise during the declutter process.

By using the techniques described in the previous chapters, it is possible to clear out up to 80 percent of the items in the home, and this can be achieved with relatively little anxiety. The aim of this book has been to present a compassionate and effective guide to help the most compulsive hoarder get their behaviors under control. And, more than simply the hoarding behaviors, it's imperative to address the underlying psychological issues that lead to hoarding in the first place. Toward that end, the previous chapters have described the variety of treatment options available to those who suffer as hoarders.

Among the most effective therapies available for hoarding disorder is cognitive-behavioral therapy. There are multiple goals of CBT, including understanding the root of hoarding behavior, utilizing techniques like motivational interviews to help them understand the discrepancy between their ideals and their real life experience. It aims to inspire change by allowing them to recognize that they are not living the life they want to live. And, once inspired, CBT can offer training in skills that are required for problem-solving and decision-making that many hoarders lack. With these skills, the hoarder will develop a greater ability to challenge their beliefs about their possessions, and that will allow them to assess their accuracy and make more appropriate decisions related to the object. Finally, for those hoarders who suffer severe anxiety during the declutter process, there are medications available to help alleviate those fears. Additionally, there are antidepressants that can help treat depression frequently experienced during the declutter process.

It is imperative to be patient in the decluttering process since the real work of the treatment is to address the underlying psychological issues. That's what will ultimately offer long-term relief. Following these guidelines will give hoarders and their loved ones the strategies they need to begin that journey of healing. This condition can be conquered, but it does take time, patience, and ongoing therapy to make progress. There are many people who have successfully made that journey using the strategies described in this book. It is possible to reclaim your life or help a loved one conquer this debilitating problem. The key is to stay positive, work the plan, don't be discouraged by setbacks, and keep moving forward. Anyone can benefit from these techniques. Really, it's about re-organizing your thoughts as much as your environment. There's no time like the present to get started on this difficult but rewarding journey. These techniques will help you regain the control you once had over your life and your environment. Get started implementing them today and get ready to say goodbye to the shame, the guilt, and the isolation this condition has caused. Say hello to your friends, your family, and your new organized, clean life.

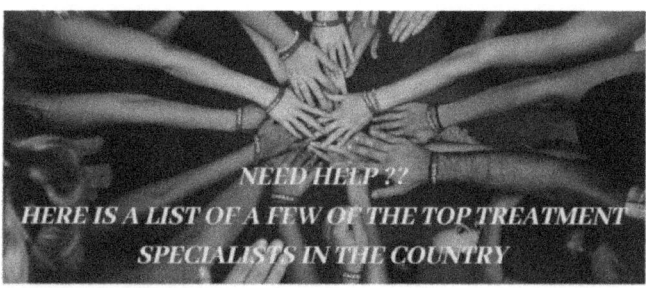

THE LIST INCLUDES:

- *Nationally renowned treatment providers*
- *One-click linked portal access*
- *Locations and contact information*
- *Things to remember when seeking or providing help*

It's one thing to need help, and another to know where to go......

To receive your Renowned Treatment List, visit the link:

<u>Renowned Treatment List</u>

REFERENCES

ADAA. (n.d.). Hoarding: The Basics | Anxiety and Depression Association of America, ADAA. Retrieved April 8, 2020, from https://adaa.org/understanding-anxiety/obsessive-compulsive-disorder-ocd/hoarding-basics

AFIC Admin. (2018, December 30). What's The Difference Between Hoarding and Collecting? Retrieved April 17, 2020, from https://www.aifc.com.au/whats-the-difference-between-collecting-and-hoarding/

American Psychiatric Association. (n.d.). What Is Hoarding Disorder? Retrieved April 2, 2020, from https://www.psychiatry.org/patients-families/hoarding-disorder/what-is-hoarding-disorder

Anxiety Canada. (n.d.). Hoarding Disorder | Here to Help. Retrieved April 13, 2020, from https://www.heretohelp.bc.ca/factsheet/hoarding-disorder

Anxiety Canada. (2019a, April 17). Challenge Negative Thinking. Retrieved April 13, 2020, from https://www.anxietycanada.com/articles/challenge-negative-thinking/

Anxiety Canada. (2019b, August 26). Helpful Thinking. Retrieved April 13, 2020, from https://www.anxietycanada.com/articles/helpful-thinking/

Ayers, C. R., Wetherell, J. L., Golshan, S., & Saxena, S. (2011). Cognitive-behavioral therapy for geriatric compulsive hoarding. *Behaviour Research and Therapy*, *49*(10), 689–694. https://doi.org/10.1016/j.brat.2011.07.002

Birchall, E., & Cronkwright, S. (2019, October 14). The Top 3 Hoarding Life Cycle Patterns: Is it true that people who hoard can't discard? Retrieved April 17, 2020, from https://www.psychologytoday.com/us/blog/conquer-the-clutter/201910/the-top-3-hoarding-life-cycle-patterns

Bowen, A. (2019, August 19). When things become too much: How to help a hoarder. Retrieved April 13, 2020, from https://www.chicagotribune.com/lifestyles/health/sc-how-to-help-a-hoarder-health-0222-20170217-story.html

Budget Dumpster. (2020, November 4). How to Declutter Your Home: A Ridiculously Thorough Guide | Budget Dumpster. Retrieved April 11, 2020, from https://www.budgetdumpster.com/resources/how-to-declutter-your-home.php

Clear, J. (2018, June 2). How to Stop Procrastinating by Using the '2-Minute Rule' Retrieved April 11, 2020, from https://medium.com/the-mission/how-to-stop-procrastinating-by-using-the-2-minute-rule-310fa8495fb9

Clear, J. C. (2019, February 1). How the 2-minute rule can help you beat procrastination and start new habits. Retrieved April 11, 2020, from https://www.cnbc.com/2019/02/01/the-2-minute-rule-how-to-stop-procrastinating-and-start-new-habits.html

Cleveland Clinic. (n.d.). Hoarding Disorder Management and Treatment. Retrieved April 11, 2020, from https://my.clevelandclinic.org/health/diseases/17682-hoarding-disorder/management-and-treatment

Cuncic, A. (2018, November 16). Understanding Cognitive Restructuring Core Part of Cognitive Behavioral Therapy. Retrieved April 11, 2020, from https://www.verywellmind.com/what-is-cognitive-restructuring-3024490

Firestone, L. (2018, October 18). Thinking Positively: Why You Need to Wire Your Brain to Think Positive. Retrieved April 13, 2020, from https://www.psychalive.org/thinking-positively/

Fitzpatrick, M., Nedeljkovic, M., Abbott, J.-A., Kyrios, M., & Moulding, R. (2018). "Blended" therapy: The development and pilot evaluation of an internet-facilitated cognitive behavioral intervention to supplement face-to-face therapy for hoarding disorder. *Internet Interventions*, *12*, 16–25. https://doi.org/10.1016/j.invent.2018.02.006

Fortin, C., & Quilici, K. (2018, April 3). 9 Ways to Create a Realistic Plan to Declutter Your Home—And Stick to It. Retrieved April 12, 2020, from https://www.workingmother.com/9-ways-to-create-realistic-plan-to-declutter-your-home-and-stick-to-it#page-2

Golden, D. (2019, November 19). How to Overcome Hoarding. Retrieved April 13, 2020, from https://www.therecoveryvillage.com/mental-health/hoarding/related/how-to-overcome-hoarding/#gref

Grisham, J., & Baldwin, P. (2015). Neuropsychological and neurophysiological insights into hoarding disorder. *Neuropsychiatric Disease and Treatment*, 951. https://doi.org/10.2147/ndt.s62084

Grohol, J. M. (2009, October 26). Why "Sleeping on It" Helps. Retrieved April 13, 2020, from https://www.livescience.com/5820-sleeping-helps.html

Henry, A. (2019, July 12). Productivity 101: An Introduction to The Pomodoro Technique. Retrieved April 11, 2020, from https://lifehacker.com/productivity-101-a-primer-to-the-pomodoro-technique-1598992730

Holt, L. (2018, August 12). Downsizing and letting go of family memorabilia. Retrieved April 13, 2020, from https://www.lindaholtcreative.com/2018/08/downsizing-and-letting-go-of-family-memorabilia/

International OCD Foundation. (2020, February 19). Treatment of HD – Cognitive Behavioral Therapy (CBT). Retrieved April 17, 2020, from https://hoarding.iocdf.org/professionals/treatment-of-hd-cognitive-behavioral-therapy-cbt/

Ivanov, V. Z., Enander, J., Mataix-Cols, D., Serlachius, E., Månsson, K. N. T., Andersson, G., ... Rück, C. (2018). Enhancing group cognitive-behavioral therapy for hoarding disorder with between-session Internet-based clinician support: A feasibility study. *Journal of Clinical Psychology*, *74*(7), 1092–1105. https://doi.org/10.1002/jclp.22589

Kane, A. C. (2019, December 13). How to Make a Vision Board. Retrieved April 11, 2020, from https://christinekane.com/how-to-make-a-vision-board/

Larkin, E. (2019, May 15). How to Stop Hoarding Before It Starts. Retrieved April 13, 2020, from https://www.thespruce.com/6-quick-tips-to-control-clutter-and-stop-hoarding-2648657

Mayo Clinic. (2018a, February 3). Hoarding disorder - Diagnosis and treatment - Mayo Clinic. Retrieved April 11, 2020, from https://www.mayoclinic.org/diseases-conditions/hoarding-disorder/diagnosis-treatment/drc-20356062

Mayo Clinic. (2018b, February 3). Hoarding disorder - Symptoms and causes. Retrieved April 12, 2020, from https://www.mayoclinic.org/diseases-conditions/hoarding-disorder/symptoms-causes/syc-20356056

NHS website. (2018, October 3). Hoarding disorder. Retrieved April 8, 2020, from https://www.nhs.uk/conditions/hoarding-disorder/

Oppong, T. (2018, June 21). The Neuroscience of Change: How to Train Your Brain to Create Better Habits. Retrieved April 13, 2020, from https://medium.com/swlh/to-break-bad-habits-you-really-have-to-change-your-brain-the-neuroscience-of-change-da735de9afdf

Owen, K. (2020, January 20). Compulsive Hoarding Treatment. Retrieved April 11, 2020, from https://www.verywellmind.com/hoarding-treatment-2510619

Phillips, A. (2017, September 3). The Psychological Benefits of Writing Things Down. Retrieved April 11, 2020, from https://rubyconnection.com.au/insights/lifestyle/the-psychological-benefits-of-writing-things-down

Rider, E. (2015, January 12). The Reason Vision Boards Work and How to Make One. Retrieved April 11, 2020, from https://www.huffpost.com/entry/the-scientific-reason-why_b_6392274

Shaw, A. M., Timpano, K. R., Steketee, G., Tolin, D. F., & Frost, R. O. (2015). Hoarding and emotional reactivity: The link between negative emotional reactions and hoarding symptomatology. *Journal of Psychiatric Research*, *63*, 84–90. https://doi.org/10.1016/j.jpsychires.2015.02.009

Staff at Oprah.com. (2018, January 2). The Best Decluttering Advice We've Heard. Retrieved April 13, 2020, from https://www.huffpost.com/entry/the-best-decluttering-advice-weve-heard_n_5a0c8906e4b0b17ffce1ffb8

Step by Step Declutter. (n.d.). Setting Goals. Retrieved April 11, 2020, from https://www.step-by-step-declutter.com/setting-goals.html

The Oprah Winfrey Show: The Podcast. (2009, October 6). 12 Tips to Overcome Hoarding. Retrieved April 13, 2020, from https://www.oprah.com/home/how-to-overcome-hoarding/all

The Recovery Village. (2020, January 27). Hoarding Statistics. Retrieved April 2, 2020, from https://www.therecoveryvillage.com/mental-health/hoarding/related/hoarding-statistics/#gref

Tolin, D. F., Hallion, L. S., Wootton, B. M., Levy, H. C., Billingsley, A. L., Das, A., … Stevens, M. C. (2018). Subjective cognitive function in hoarding disorder. *Psychiatry Research*, *265*, 215–220. https://doi.org/10.1016/j.psychres.2018.05.003

Vandenberg, S. (2019, July 1). How to clean a hoarder's house - Hoarding cleaning tips and steps. Retrieved April 12, 2020, from https://www.servicemastersanfrancisco.com/clean-hoarders-house/

Weir, K. (2020, April 1). Treating people with hoarding disorder. Retrieved April 17, 2020, from https://www.apa.org/monitor/2020/04/ce-corner-hoarding

Woods, R. (2020, November 4). How to Declutter Your

Home: A Ridiculously Thorough Guide | Budget Dumpster. Retrieved April 11, 2020, from https://www.budgetdumpster.com/resources/how-to-declutter-your-home.php

Yap, K., Eppingstall, J., Brennan, C., Le, B., & Grisham, J. R. (2020). Emotional attachment to objects mediates the relationship between loneliness and hoarding symptoms. *Journal of Obsessive-Compulsive and Related Disorders, 24,* 100487. https://doi.org/10.1016/j.jocrd.2019.100487

www.ingramcontent.com/pod-product-compliance
Lightning Source LLC
Chambersburg PA
CBHW031156020426
42333CB00013B/688

9781952817014